# Atrial Fibrillation in Heart Failure

*Editors*

BENJAMIN A. STEINBERG
JONATHAN P. PICCINI Sr

# CARDIOLOGY CLINICS

www.cardiology.theclinics.com

May 2019 • Volume 37 • Number 2

**ELSEVIER**

1600 John F. Kennedy Boulevard • Suite 1800 • Philadelphia, Pennsylvania, 19103-2899

http://www.theclinics.com

**CARDIOLOGY CLINICS Volume 37, Number 2**
**May 2019 ISSN 0733-8651, ISBN-13: 978-0-323-67854-4**

Editor: Stacy Eastman
Developmental Editor: Laura Kavanaugh

*Cardiology Clinics* (ISSN 0733-8651) is published quarterly by Elsevier Inc., 360 Park Avenue South, New York, NY 10010-1710. Months of issue are February, May, August, and November. Business and Editorial Offices: 1600 John F. Kennedy Blvd., Ste. 1800, Philadelphia, PA 19103-2899. Customer Service Office: 3251 Riverport Lane, Maryland Heights, MO 63043. Periodicals postage paid at New York, NY and additional mailing offices. Subscription prices are $349.00 per year for US individuals, $672.00 per year for US institutions, $100.00 per year for US students and residents, $432.00 per year for Canadian individuals, $843.00 per year for Canadian institutions, $466.00 per year for international individuals, $843.00 per year for international institutions and $220.00 per year for Canadian and international students/residents. To receive student/resident rate, orders must be accompanied by name of affiliated institution, data of term, and the *signature* of program/residency coordinator on institution letterhead. Orders will be billed at individual rate until proof of status is received. Foreign air speed delivery is included in all *Clinics* subscription prices. All prices are subject to change without notice. **POSTMASTER:** Send address changes to *Cardiology Clinics*, Elsevier Health Sciences Division, Subscription Customer Service, 3251 Riverport Lane, Maryland Heights, MO 63043. **Customer Service: 1-800-654-2452 (U.S. and Canada); 314-447-8871 (outside U.S. and Canada). Fax: 314-447-8029. E-mail: journalscustomerservice-usa@ elsevier.com (for print support); journalsonlinesupport-usa@elsevier.com (for online support).**

*Reprints.* For copies of 100 or more, of articles in this publication, please contact the Commercial Reprints Department, Elsevier Inc. 360 Park Avenue South, New York, NY 10010-1710. Tel.: 212-633-3874; Fax: 212-633-3820; E-mail: reprints@elsevier.com.

*Cardiology Clinics* is also published in Spanish by McGraw-Hill Interamericana Editores S. A., P.O. Box 5-237, 06500, Mexico D F., Mexico; in Portuguese by Reichmann and Alfonso Editores Rio de Janeiro, Brazil; and in Greek by Dimitrios P. Lagos, 8 Pondon Street, GR115-28 Ilissia, Greece.

*Cardiology Clinics* is covered in *MEDLINE/PubMed (Index Medicus), Excerpta Medica, The Cumulative Index to Nursing and Allied Health Literature* (CINAHL).

# Contributors

## EDITORIAL BOARD

**JORDAN M. PRUTKIN, MD, MHS, FHRS**
Assistant Professor of Medicine, Division of
Cardiology/Electrophysiology, UW Medical
Center, Seattle, Washington, USA

**DAVID M. SHAVELLE, MD, FACC, FSCAI**
Associate Professor, Keck School of
Medicine of USC, Director, General
Cardiovascular Fellowship Program,
Director, Cardiac Catheterization
Laboratory, LAC + USC Medical Center,
Division of Cardiovascular Medicine,
University of Southern California,
Los Angeles, California, USA

**TERRENCE D. WELCH, MD, FACC**
Assistant Professor, Department of
Medicine, Section of Cardiology,
Dartmouth-Hitchcock Medical Center,
Lebanon, New Hampshire, USA;
Department of Internal Medicine, Dartmouth
Geisel School of Medicine, Hanover,
New Hampshire, USA

**AUDREY H. WU, MD**
Assistant Professor, Internal Medicine,
University of Michigan, Ann Arbor, Michigan,
USA

## EDITORS

**BENJAMIN A. STEINBERG, MD, MHS,
FACC, FHRS**
Division of Cardiovascular Medicine, University
of Utah Health Sciences Center, Salt Lake City,
Utah, USA

**JONATHAN P. PICCINI Sr, MD, MHS, FACC,
FAHA, FHRS**
Duke Center for Atrial Fibrillation,
Duke University Hospital, Duke Clinical
Research Institute, Durham, North Carolina,
USA

## AUTHORS

**KIA AFSHAR, MD**
Intermountain Medical Center Heart Institute,
Murray, Utah, USA; Department of Internal
Medicine, University of Utah, Salt Lake City,
Utah, USA

**PRADYUMNA AGASTHI, MD**
Cardiology Fellow, Department of
Cardiovascular Diseases, Mayo Clinic,
Phoenix, Arizona, USA

**RAMI ALHARETHI, MD**
Intermountain Medical Center Heart Institute,
Murray, Utah, USA; Department of Internal
Medicine, University of Utah, Salt Lake City,
Utah, USA

**EMELIA J. BENJAMIN, MD, FACC, FAHA**
Professor of Medicine and Epidemiology,
Evans Department of Medicine,
Cardiovascular Medicine Section,
Boston University School of Medicine,
Department of Epidemiology, Boston
University School of Public Health,
Boston, Massachusetts, USA;
The Framingham Heart Study,
Framingham, Massachusetts,
USA

**RAHUL BHARDWAJ, MD**
Loma Linda University, Loma Linda, California,
USA

**T. JARED BUNCH, MD**
Intermountain Medical Center Heart Institute, Intermountain Heart Rhythm Specialists, Intermountain Medical Center, Eccles Outpatient Care Center, Murray, Utah, USA; Department of Internal Medicine, Stanford University, Palo Alto, California, USA

**JOHN D. DAY, MD**
Intermountain Medical Center Heart Institute, Murray, Utah, USA

**CHRISTOPHER V. DᴇSIMONE, MD, PhD**
Department of Cardiovascular Diseases, Mayo Clinic, Rochester, Minnesota, USA

**MAJD A. EL-HARASIS, MBBS**
Division of Internal Medicine, Mayo Clinic, Rochester, Minnesota, USA

**CHRISTOPHER R. ELLIS, MD, FACC, FHRS**
Associate Professor of Medicine, Director Left Atrial Appendage Program, Vanderbilt University Medical Center, Nashville, Tennessee, USA

**DEEPA M. GOPAL, MD, MS**
Assistant Professor of Medicine, Evans Department of Medicine, Cardiovascular Medicine Section, Boston University School of Medicine, Boston, Massachusetts, USA

**COLLEEN HANLEY, MD**
Cardiac Electrophysiologist, Lankenau Heart Institute, Wynnewood, Pennsylvania, USA

**ROBERT H. HELM, MD, FHRS**
Assistant Professor of Medicine, Evans Department of Medicine, Cardiovascular Medicine Section, Boston University School of Medicine, Boston, Massachusetts, USA

**ARVINDH N. KANAGASUNDRAM, MD, FHRS**
Assistant Professor of Medicine, Vanderbilt University Medical Center, Nashville, Tennessee, USA

**ANKUR A. KARNIK, MD, FHRS, FACC**
Assistant Professor of Medicine, Evans Department of Medicine, Cardiovascular Medicine Section, Boston University School of Medicine, Boston, Massachusetts, USA

**DAVID M. KAYE, MBBS, PhD**
Department of Clinical Research, The Baker Heart and Diabetes Institute, Department of Cardiology, The Alfred Hospital, Melbourne, Victoria, Australia; Department of Medicine, Monash University, Clayton, Victoria, Australia

**AMANULLA KHAJI, MD**
Clinical Cardiac Electrophysiology Fellow, Lankenau Heart Institute, Wynnewood, Pennsylvania, USA

**PETER M. KISTLER, MBBS, PhD**
Department of Clinical Research, The Baker Heart and Diabetes Institute, Department of Cardiology, The Alfred Hospital, Melbourne, Victoria, Australia; Department of Medicine, The University of Melbourne, Parkville, Victoria, Australia

**DARAE KO, MD, MSc**
Evans Department of Medicine, Cardiovascular Medicine Section, Boston University School of Medicine, Boston, Massachusetts, USA

**JACOB S. KORUTH, MD**
Director, Experimental Lab, Assistant Professor of Medicine, Leona M. and Harvey B. Helmsley Electrophysiology Center, Mount Sinai Medical Center, New York, New York, USA

**PETER R. KOWEY, MD, FACC, FHRS, FAHA**
Chairman Emeritus of Cardiology, Lankenau Heart Institute, Professor of Medicine and Clinical Pharmacology, Jefferson Medical College, Philadelphia, Pennsylvania, USA

**JUSTIN Z. LEE, MBBS**
Cardiology Fellow, Department of Cardiovascular Diseases, Mayo Clinic, Phoenix, Arizona, USA

**LIANG-HAN LING, MBBS, PhD**
Department of Clinical Research, The Baker Heart and Diabetes Institute, Department of Cardiology, The Alfred Hospital, Melbourne, Victoria, Australia; Department of Medicine, The University of Melbourne, Parkville, Victoria, Australia

**ZAK LORING, MD**
Cardiology Fellow, Division of Cardiology, Section of Electrophysiology, Duke University Medical Center, Duke Clinical Research Institute, Durham, North Carolina, USA

**HEIDI T. MAY, PhD**
Intermountain Medical Center Heart Institute, Murray, Utah, USA

**SIVA K. MULPURU, MD**
Associate Professor, Department of Cardiovascular Diseases, Mayo Clinic, Rochester, Minnesota, USA

**SHANE NANAYAKKARA, MBBS**
Department of Clinical Research, The Baker Heart and Diabetes Institute, Department of Cardiology, The Alfred Hospital, Melbourne, Victoria, Australia; Department of Medicine, Monash University, Clayton, Victoria, Australia

**PETER A. NOSEWORTHY, MD**
Department of Cardiovascular Diseases, Robert D. and Patricia E. Kern Center for the Science of Health Care Delivery, Mayo Clinic, Rochester, Minnesota, USA

**JONATHAN P. PICCINI Sr, MD, MHS, FACC, FAHA, FHRS**
Duke Center for Atrial Fibrillation, Duke University Hospital, Duke Clinical Research Institute, Durham, North Carolina, USA

**SANDEEP PRABHU, MBBS, PhD**
Department of Clinical Research, The Baker Heart and Diabetes Institute, Department of Cardiology, The Alfred Hospital, Melbourne, Victoria, Australia; Department of Cardiology, Royal Melbourne Hospital, Department of Medicine, The University of Melbourne, Parkville, Victoria, Australia

**RAVI RANJAN, MD, PhD**
Associate Professor, Division of Cardiovascular Medicine, Department of Internal Medicine, Nora Eccles Harrison Cardiovascular Research and Training Institute, Department of Biomedical Engineering, University of Utah, Salt Lake City, Utah, USA

**PRASHANTHAN SANDERS, MBBS, PhD**
Director of Cardiac Electrophysiology, Department of Cardiology, Royal Adelaide Hospital, Director of the Centre for Heart Rhythm Disorders, University of Adelaide, Adelaide, Australia

**BENJAMIN A. STEINBERG, MD, MHS, FACC, FHRS**
Division of Cardiovascular Medicine, University of Utah Health Sciences Center, Salt Lake City, Utah, USA

**MICHAEL B. STOKES, MBBS**
Cardiologist, Department of Cardiology, Royal Adelaide Hospital, PhD Candidate, University of Adelaide, Adelaide, Australia

**HARIHARAN SUGUMAR, MBBS**
Department of Clinical Research, The Baker Heart and Diabetes Institute, Department of Cardiology, The Alfred Hospital, Melbourne, Victoria, Australia; Department of Cardiology, Royal Melbourne Hospital, Department of Medicine, The University of Melbourne, Parkville, Victoria, Australia

**ALBERT Y. SUN, MD**
Assistant Professor of Medicine, Division of Cardiology, Section of Electrophysiology, Duke University Medical Center, Division of Cardiology, Section of Electrophysiology, Durham VA Medical Center, Durham, North Carolina, USA

**MARIA TERRICABRAS, MD**
Southlake Regional Health Centre, University of Toronto, Newmarket, Ontario, Canada

**ANDREW TSENG, MD**
Resident, Department of Internal Medicine, Mayo Clinic, Phoenix, Arizona, USA

**ATUL VERMA, MD, FRCPC, FHRS**
Southlake Regional Health Centre, University of Toronto, Newmarket, Ontario, Canada

**ALEKSANDR VOSKOBOINIK, MBBS**
Department of Clinical Research, The Baker Heart and Diabetes Institute, Department of Cardiology, The Alfred Hospital, Melbourne, Victoria, Australia; Department of Cardiology, Royal Melbourne Hospital, Department of Medicine, The University of Melbourne, Parkville, Victoria, Australia

**KENNOSUKE YAMASHITA, MD, PhD**
Division of Cardiovascular Medicine,
Department of Internal Medicine, Nora Eccles
Harrison Cardiovascular Research and
Training Institute, University of Utah, Salt Lake
City, Utah, USA

**XIAOXI YAO, PhD**
Division of Health Care Policy and Research,
Department of Health Sciences Research,
Robert D. and Patricia E. Kern Center for the
Science of Health Care Delivery, Mayo Clinic,
Rochester, Minnesota, USA

# Contents

**Preface: Atrial Fibrillation and Heart Failure: In This Challenge Lies Opportunity**    xiii

Benjamin A. Steinberg and Jonathan P. Piccini Sr

**Epidemiology of Atrial Fibrillation and Heart Failure: A Growing and Important Problem**    119

Ankur A. Karnik, Deepa M. Gopal, Darae Ko, Emelia J. Benjamin, and Robert H. Helm

The global prevalence of atrial fibrillation (AF) and heart failure (HF) is rising. Population-based studies have observed that AF and HF often coexist, predispose to each other, and share risk factors. Age is the most potent risk factor for both AF and HF, but race plays an important role. Although AF and HF share common risk factors, adjusting for these risk factors does not explain the higher risk of AF patients developing HF and vice versa. Common pathophysiologic mechanisms may explain this linkage. The morbidity and mortality outcomes with combined AF and HF are substantial and warrant improved preventive strategies.

**Pathophysiology of Atrial Fibrillation and Heart Failure: Dangerous Interactions**    131

Hariharan Sugumar, Shane Nanayakkara, Sandeep Prabhu, Aleksandr Voskoboinik, David M. Kaye, Liang-Han Ling, and Peter M. Kistler

Atrial fibrillation and heart failure (HF) frequently coexist and are associated with a significant increase in morbidity and mortality. Despite the shared common risk factors atrial fibrillation and HF subtypes exacerbate each other. This review provides an overview of the pathophysiologic relationship between atrial fibrillation and the two most common types of heart failure syndromes: HF with reduced ejection fraction and HF with preserved ejection fraction.

**Tackling Patient-Reported Outcomes in Atrial Fibrillation and Heart Failure: Identifying Disease-Specific Symptoms?**    139

Benjamin A. Steinberg and Jonathan P. Piccini Sr

Atrial fibrillation (AF) and heart failure (HF) both significantly affect morbidity and mortality and also account for high symptom burden and impaired health-related quality of life (hrQoL). Several well-designed and broadly implemented patient-reported outcome instruments are available for both AF and HF and can easily measure hrQoL in each disease process. A better understanding of the diverse phenotypes of AF and HF, as well as the heterogeneous treatment effects of disease-specific interventions, is necessary to further disentangle the complex relationship between symptoms of AF and HF.

**Imaging for Risk Stratification in Atrial Fibrillation with Heart Failure**    147

Kennosuke Yamashita and Ravi Ranjan

Atrial fibrillation (AF) is the most common cardiac rhythm disorder and is associated with heart failure (HF). Cardiac imaging modalities play an important role in risk assessment and managing AF. This article reviews the use of cardiac imaging for risk assessment and to optimize treatment strategy in patients with AF and HF. First, the clinical role of echocardiography, computed tomography, and cardiac magnetic resonance for risk stratification is provided. Second, the value of imaging in catheter ablation is reviewed, including preoperative assessment, optimizing patient selection for ablation, use during the ablation procedure, and postoperative scar assessment.

### Does Left Ventricular Systolic Function Matter? Treating Atrial Fibrillation in HFrEF Versus HFpEF    157

Michael B. Stokes and Prashanthan Sanders

Atrial fibrillation (AF) and heart failure (HF) pose international health care challenges that contribute significantly to hospitalizations, morbidity, mortality, and significant health care costs. Both AF and HF contribute to the development of each other and both are associated with a worsened prognosis when they occur together. Assessment of systolic function via transthoracic echocardiography is essential in the investigation of the AF patient. Clinical and echocardiographic assessment may classify AF patients with HF into HF with reduced ejection fraction (HF-rEF) and HF with preserved ejection fraction (HF-pEF). Such classification can assist in numerous important management decisions in AF.

### Randomized Clinical Trials of Catheter Ablation of Atrial Fibrillation in Congestive Heart Failure: Knowns and Unmet Needs    167

Maria Terricabras, Jonathan P. Piccini Sr, and Atul Verma

Atrial fibrillation (AF) and heart failure (HF) are conditions that frequently coexist and are associated with worse outcomes compared with either condition alone. Although rhythm control with antiarrhythmic drug treatment is not superior to rate control in this population, catheter ablation has emerged as an alternative and more effective treatment of maintenance of sinus rhythm. Some trials have shown benefit in hospitalization and mortality, but additional studies are needed. The authors summarize the current evidence regarding catheter ablation outcomes, efficacy, and safety and discuss the unmet needs of the existing and ongoing randomized clinical trials.

### Mechanisms of Improved Mortality Following Ablation: Does Ablation Restore Beta-Blocker Benefit in Atrial Fibrillation/Heart Failure?    177

T. Jared Bunch, Heidi T. May, Kia Afshar, Rami Alharethi, and John D. Day

Observational trials have shown that atrial fibrillation ablation favorably impacts long-term outcomes in systolic heart failure. These outcomes have been confirmed by randomized prospective trials highlighting the favorable impact of ablation on left ventricular function and remodeling, risk of heart failure hospitalization, and mortality. Ablation along with established heart failure medications is new and supported conceptually by the value of restoring sinus rhythm, avoiding long-term antiarrhythmic drugs, and minimizing drug–drug interactions. Observational data suggest a potential long-term benefit of beta-blockers with ablation that becomes augmented as follow-up is extended from 1 to 5 years.

### Atrial Fibrillation Ablation Should Be First-line Therapy in Patients with Heart Failure Reduced Ejection Fraction    185

Pradyumna Agasthi, Andrew Tseng, Justin Z. Lee, and Siva K. Mulpuru

Catheter ablation for atrial fibrillation in patients with heart failure with reduced ejection fraction is associated with improvement in patient-centered outcomes, such as mortality, heart failure readmission, and atrial fibrillation recurrence, compared with standard medical therapy with or without device therapy. The evidence is not as robust in patients with atrial fibrillation and heart failure with preserved ejection fraction.

## Atrial Fibrillation Ablation Should Be First-Line Therapy in Heart Failure Patients: CON

197

Amanulla Khaji, Colleen Hanley, and Peter R. Kowey

Heart failure (HF) and atrial fibrillation (AF) are the epidemics of the twenty-first century. These often coexist and are the cause of major morbidity and mortality. Management of these patients has posed a significant challenge to the medical community. Guideline-directed pharmacologic therapy for heart failure is important; however, there is no clear consensus on how best to treat AF with concomitant HF. In this article, we provide an in-depth review of the management of AF in patients with HF and provide insight as to why catheter ablation should not be the first line of therapy in this population.

## Novel Ablation Approaches for Challenging Atrial Fibrillation Cases (Mapping, Irrigation, and Catheters)

207

Rahul Bhardwaj and Jacob S. Koruth

Catheter ablation for atrial fibrillation has improved in part due to advances in technology and techniques. Improved power delivery through contact force and irrigation and new balloon-based catheter systems for pulmonary vein isolation have resulted in greater success in paroxysmal atrial fibrillation. New tools are under development to facilitate understanding targets for ablation in persistent atrial fibrillation and create permanent ablation lesions safely and quickly.

## Prediction and Management of Recurrences after Catheter Ablation in Atrial Fibrillation and Heart Failure

221

Majd A. El-Harasis, Christopher V. DeSimone, Xiaoxi Yao, and Peter A. Noseworthy

Catheter ablation is recommended in patients with symptomatic atrial fibrillation (AF) refractory to pharmacologic therapy. AF recurrence is common postablation, particularly in patients with heart failure, because of multiple structural and functional changes that can occur. Determining predictors of AF recurrence has become increasingly important. These include increased left atrial volume, termination of AF during the index ablation, electrocardiogram parameters, and serum biomarkers. Cardiac MRI can also determine the degree of scarring and left atrial sphericity, which is used in risk prediction scores. In patients with recurrence, further treatment options include pharmacologic therapy and atrioventricular nodal ablation with pacing.

## Should His Bundle Pacing Be Preferred over Cardiac Resynchronization Therapy Following Atrioventricular Junction Ablation?

231

Zak Loring and Albert Y. Sun

Atrial fibrillation (AF) and heart failure (HF) are associated with high morbidity and mortality, which is particularly detrimental when patients develop rapid ventricular rates (RVR). Atrioventricular junction (AVJ) ablation with pacemaker implantation has been used as a method of achieving rate control in patients with incessant AF with RVR. Right ventricular only pacing is known to be harmful in the setting of HF. His bundle pacing (HBP) and biventricular (BiV) pacing both offer durable pacing solutions that offer more physiologic activation. This review describes the benefits and drawbacks of HBP and BiV pacing in HF patients after AVJ ablation.

**Atrial Fibrillation in Heart Failure: Left Atrial Appendage Management**          **241**

Christopher R. Ellis and Arvindh N. Kanagasundram

Atrial fibrillation is common in patients with congestive heart failure (CHF). Due to reduced left atrial appendage (LAA) emptying velocities and increased sludge formation, a higher rate of stroke and embolism are seen with CHF. Up to 50% of CHF patients are inadequately covered for stroke protection with anticoagulation, and, even while on therapy, CHF patients are at risk for failure to clear LAA or left ventricular (LV) thrombus. Device-based LAA closure (LAAC) alternatives exist. Following intracardiac device closure, an increased rate of device-related thrombus is seen in heart failure patients, which warrants further study to optimize LAAC benefits.

# CARDIOLOGY CLINICS

**FORTHCOMING ISSUES**

*August 2019*
**Diabetes/Kidney/Heart Disease**
Silvi Shah and Charuhas V. Thakar, *Editors*

*November 2019*
**Cardio-Oncology**
Monika Jacquelina Leja, *Editor*

*February 2020*
**Aortic Valve Disease**
Marie-Annick Clavel and Philippe Pibarot,
*Editors*

**RECENT ISSUES**

*February 2019*
**Hypertrophic Cardiomyopathy**
Srihari S. Naidu and Julio A. Panza, *Editors*

*November 2018*
**Mechanical Circulatory Support**
Palak Shah and Jennifer A. Cowger, *Editors*

*August 2018*
**Resuscitation**
Andrew M. McCoy, *Editor*

---

SERIES OF RELATED INTEREST

*Cardiac Electrophysiology Clinics*
*Heart Failure Clinics*
*Interventional Cardiology Clinics*

---

**THE CLINICS ARE AVAILABLE ONLINE!**
Access your subscription at:
www.theclinics.com

# Preface
# Atrial Fibrillation and Heart Failure: In This Challenge Lies Opportunity

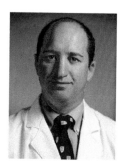 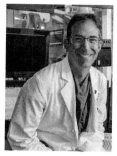

Benjamin A. Steinberg, MD, MHS, FACC, FHRS　　Jonathan P. Piccini Sr, MD, MHS, FACC, FAHA, FHRS

*Editors*

The last century of cardiovascular research and care has seen dramatic reductions in disease burden, specifically of ischemic heart disease and related events. This has been an unquestionable success for the medical community and has improved the lives of millions of patients. With these improved treatments of primarily atherothrombotic processes, we have entered a new phase of cardiovascular disease where longevity-altering acute coronary syndromes are instead chronically managed, yielding a burgeoning population of downstream cardiovascular disease. The combined effects of dramatic improvements in atherothrombotic cardiovascular disease management, coupled with naturally aging populations, particularly in the United States, is giving rise to new epidemics: record rates of atrial fibrillation (AF) and heart failure (HF). This is not a coincidence; advanced age and underlying structural heart disease are both potent risk factors for AF and HF, which may develop sequentially, or coincidentally. Among patients with both AF and HF, the combination of the two is worse than the sum of the parts: patients with both AF and HF tend to feel particularly poorly and have a particularly high risk for adverse clinical events. In this challenge lies opportunity, the management of patients with AF and HF presents new prospects for reducing morbidity and mortality, while developing new, disease-altering approaches and therapies.

In this issue of *Cardiology Clinics*, we present a series of articles by world-renowned experts in their fields, in an effort to encapsulate the current states of the challenges, successes, and future developments in managing patients with AF and HF. You will find comprehensive discussion of the epidemiology of this challenging problem, the dynamic and overlapping nature of pathophysiology, implications for management, treatment challenges, and opportunities to successfully manage these patients now and in the future. In the end, we hope you will come away with an appreciation for the severity of the problem, a paradigm for management of these high-risk patients, and optimism for the future of treating atrial fibrillation and heart failure.

Benjamin A. Steinberg, MD, MHS, FACC, FHRS
Division of Cardiovascular Medicine
University of Utah Health Sciences Center
30 North 1900 East, Room 4A100
Salt Lake City, UT 84132, USA

Jonathan P. Piccini Sr, MD, MHS, FACC, FAHA, FHRS
Duke Center for Atrial Fibrillation
Duke University Hospital and
Duke Clinical Research Institute
PO Box 17969
Durham, NC 27710, USA

*E-mail addresses:*
benjamin.steinberg@hsc.utah.edu
(B.A. Steinberg)
jonathan.piccini@duke.edu (J.P. Piccini)

Cardiol Clin 37 (2019) xiii
https://doi.org/10.1016/j.ccl.2019.02.001
0733-8651/19/© 2019 Published by Elsevier Inc.

cardiology.theclinics.com

# Epidemiology of Atrial Fibrillation and Heart Failure
## A Growing and Important Problem

Ankur A. Karnik, MD, FHRS[a],*, Deepa M. Gopal, MD, MS[a],
Darae Ko, MD, MSc[c], Emelia J. Benjamin, MD[a,b,c],
Robert H. Helm, MD, FHRS[a]

**KEYWORDS**

- Atrial fibrillation • Heart failure • Epidemiology • Risk factors • Prognosis

**KEY POINTS**

- Atrial fibrillation (AF) and heart failure (HF) are global epidemics that contribute substantially to cardiovascular morbidity, mortality, and health care costs.
- Most population-based cohorts are rather homogeneous but there is recognition of significant gender and racial differences in AF and HF incidence, lifetime risk, and outcomes.
- AF increases lifetime risk of HF and vice versa.
- The interaction between the two is complex. The influence of shared risk factors is hard to completely account for because they play a significant role in the pathogenesis of each other.
- Relative risk of mortality in patients with preexisting HF who develop AF is higher than in patients with preexisting AF who developed HF.

## INTRODUCTION

Atrial fibrillation (AF) and heart failure (HF) are highly prevalent and are associated with high health care costs and significant morbidity and mortality. In the year 2010, AF was estimated to affect 2.7 million to 6.1 million persons in the United States and 33.5 million persons worldwide.[1] By the year 2030, 12.1 million Americans are projected to have AF.[2] AF is associated with significant morbidity, including poor quality of life, HF, myocardial infarction,[3] dementia,[4] stroke, and death.[5,6] In the more than 50 years of follow-up of the Framingham Heart Study (FHS) , the age-adjusted prevalence of AF has increased 4-fold.[7] Hospitalizations for AF in the United States have increased 23% between 2000 and 2010,[8] with an estimated incremental cost of $26 billion in 2008.[9]

HF is also highly prevalent, affecting an estimated 6.5 million Americans greater than or equal to 20 years of age.[10] The prevalence of HF is projected to increase 46% between 2012 and 2030,

Disclosure Statement: R.H. Helm is a research support for GE Healthcare, AdreView Myocardial Imaging for Risk Evaluation 05/22/2017 to 05/21/2021 (PI). A.A. Karnik, D.M. Gopal, D. Ko, and E.J. Benjamin have nothing to disclose.
Source of Funding: This work was supported by Velux Foundation and by NIH/NHLBI 2R01HL092577 and 1R01HL128914; American Heart Association, 18SFRN34110082; 17FTF33670369 (D.M. Gopal).
[a] Evans Department of Medicine, Cardiovascular Medicine Section, Boston University School of Medicine, 72 East Harrison Street, Collamore 8, Boston, MA 02118, USA; [b] Department of Epidemiology, Boston University School of Public Health, 72 East Harrison Street, Collamore 8, Boston, MA 02118, USA; [c] The Framingham Heart Study, Framingham, MA, USA
* Corresponding author. 72 East Harrison Street, Collamore 817, Boston, MA 02118.
E-mail address: ankur.karnik@bmc.org

cardiology.theclinics.com

affecting greater than or equal to 8 million people greater than or equal to 18 years of age.[11] Over this same time period, the total cost due to HF is estimated to grow from $30.7 billion to $69.7 billion.[11] This review presents epidemiologic data on the lifetime risk, incidence, prevalence, and risk factors for AF and HF. Their temporality, causation, and joint effect on mortality are discussed.

## LIFETIME RISK
### Lifetime Risk of Atrial Fibrillation

The lifetime risk of AF has been studied in several community-based cohort studies. The FHS reported that the lifetime risk of AF in 55-year-old individuals was 37%.[12] The Atherosclerosis Risk in Communities (ARIC) study observed that the lifetime risk of AF was approximately 1 in 3 in whites and 1 in 5 in African Americans (AAs).[13] European cohort studies have shown similar risk. The BiomarCaRE (Biomarker for Cardiovascular Risk Assessment in Europe) consortium reported that one-third of men and women developed AF during their lifetime.[14] The lifetime risk of AF varies by clinical risk factor[13,15] and genetic factors and is lowest with individuals with low clinical and polygenic risk (22.4%) and highest with high clinical and polygenic risk (48.2%).[12] The polygenic risk scores were constructed from single-nucleotide polymorphism groups selected based on prior genome-wide association study of AF.[12]

### Lifetime Risk of Heart Failure

The FHS reported a lifetime risk of HF at age 40 years as 21.0% for men and 20.3% for women. In those without myocardial infarction, this risk decreased to 11.4% for men and 15.4% for women. On the other hand, the lifetime risk doubled for those with blood pressure greater than or equal to 160/100 mm Hg compared with those with blood pressure less than or equal to 140/90 mm Hg.[16] The Rotterdam Study showed somewhat higher lifetime risk in a European cohort (29% for women and 33% for men at age 55 years) but there were differences in HF criteria.[17] A pooled study of cohorts from the Chicago Heart Association Detection Project in Industry, ARIC, and Cardiovascular Health Study (CHS) was used to compare risk of HF in AAs and whites; the lifetime risk at age 45 years was 24% to 46% in AA women, 32% to 39% in white women, 20% to 29% in AA men, 30% to 42% in white men.[18] The risk was greatest in those with higher blood pressure and body mass index (BMI) across all age and racial groups. AA men had higher non–cardiovascular-related mortality, which limited lifetime risk of HF.[18]

## INFLUENCE OF AGE, GENDER, AND RACE ON RISK OF ATRIAL FIBRILLATION AND HEART FAILURE
### Age

Advancing age is the most potent risk factor for AF.[7] In the BiomarCaRE study, the incidence of AF increased significantly after age 50 years in men and age 60 years in women, although the lifetime risk of AF was similar.[14] During 50 years of observation in the FHS, age continued to be a powerful risk factor for AF. In 1998 to 2007, individuals ages 60 years to 69 years, 70 years to 79 years, and 80 years to 89 years had 4.98-fold, 7.35-fold, and 9.33-fold risks of AF, respectively, compared with those ages 50 years to 59 years.[7] Despite the powerful influence of age, the prospective Multi-Ethnic Study of Atherosclerosis (MESA) study observed that in individuals greater than 65 years of age, Hispanics, Chinese, and AAs still had significantly less AF than white individuals.[19]

Similarly, age is an important risk factor for HF. In the Rotterdam Study, the incident rate of HF increased from 1.4/1000 person-years in those ages 55 years to 59 years to 47.4/1000 person-years in those ages greater than or equal to 90 years.[17]

### Gender

The epidemiology of AF differs between men and women in North American and European populations.[20,21] Most community-based studies have shown a higher AF incidence in men. The BiomarCaRE study reported that the incidence of AF was 2.2% higher in men than women.[14] Similarly, the FHS and the Rotterdam Study showed AF incidence rates (per 1000 person-years) of 1.6 and 8.9 in women, respectively, compared with 3.8 and 11.5, respectively, in men.[7,22] AF is also more prevalent among men. Analysis of data on Medicare beneficiaries greater than or equal to 65 years of age showed a prevalence of 7.4% in women versus 10.3% in men.[23] A Scottish retrospective study of National Health Service patients found the prevalence of AF was 0.79% in women and 0.94% in men.[24] Gender differences in the distribution of risk factors for AF seem to explain higher incidence of AF in men.[25] Finally, longer life expectancy may explain why there are similar numbers of men and women with AF in the population despite women having an overall lower incidence of AF than men.[20,23]

The incidence and prevalence of HF in women differ from those in men as well. The Rotterdam Study reported HF incidence (per 1000 person-years) of 12.5 in women and 17.6 in men. Similar gender trends in HF incidence were seen in

FHS,[26] CHS,[27] and the New Haven, Connecticut, cohort of the Established Populations for Epidemiologic Studies of the Elderly program.[28] Prevalence of HF is higher in men overall. In the Olmsted County cohort, Minnesota, the prevalence of HF was 1.7% in women and 2.7% in men.[29] The Rotterdam Study also showed a higher prevalence of HF in men.[17] Regarding HF, the most substantive gender difference is that men are more likely to develop HF with reduced ejection fraction (HFrEF), whereas women are more likely to develop HF with preserved ejection fraction (HFpEF).[30]

## Race

The incidence, prevalence, and lifetime risk of AF are lower in nonwhite populations. The Healthcare Cost and Utilization Project, a hospital-based administrative data study, found a lower incidence of AF in AA, Asian, and Hispanic patients compared with whites.[31] Analysis of the MESA study revealed that overall AF incidence (1000 person-years) was significantly lower among Hispanic, AA, and Chinese participants (6.1, 5,8, and 3.9, respectively) compared with whites (11.2).[19] In the ATRIA (Anticoagulation and Risk factors in Atrial Fibrillation) study, the prevalence of AF was 2.2% in white versus 1.5% in AA participants over the age of 50.[32] The ARIC study found that AA men and women and had 41% lower age-adjusted and gender-adjusted risk of AF compared with whites after an average 15-year follow-up.[33] The National Hospital Discharge Survey/National Center for Health Statistics between 1996 and 2001 found that of patients with AF hospitalizations, 71.2% were white, 5.6% black, and 2.0% other races (20.8% were not specified).[34] The degree of European ancestry is associated with incidence of AF. Genome-wide analysis interrogating for ancestry informative markers in 19,784 participants from the CHS and ARIC studies found that every 10% increase in European ancestry increased the risk of AF by 13%.[35]

Although the AF incidence is lower in AA individuals, they have worse outcomes than their white counterparts. In ARIC, in individuals with AF, compared with whites, AAs had a 1.5-fold to 2-fold risk of stroke, HF, and death.[36]

The risk of HF also varies by race. The MESA study reported that AA participants had the highest risk of HF, followed by Hispanic, white, and Chinese participants (4.6, 3.5, 2.4, and 1.0 per 1000 person-years, respectively). AAs were most likely to have incident HF not preceded by myocardial infarction.[37] The higher risk of HF in AAs has been attributed to increased risk factor burden.[37,38] The biracial Coronary Artery Risk Development in Young Adults study also demonstrated the influence of risk factor and race on HF incidence. Of 5115 participants ages 18 years to 30 years who were followed for 20 years, 27 developed HF and all but 1 were black. Predictors for HF were higher diastolic blood pressure, higher BMI, lower HDL, and kidney disease.[39] Despite higher incidence of HF in AA, the lifetime risk was highest in white men and lowest in AA women based on the pooled data from Chicago Heart Association Detection Project, ARIC, and CHS, as discussed previously.[18]

## SHARED RISK FACTORS

AF and HF often occur in the same patients because they share common risk factors.[16,27,40,41] As reviewed previously, both conditions are associated with nonmodifiable risk factors, including increasing age, gender, and race. Other common risk factors include elevated blood pressure, obesity, obstructive sleep apnea (OSA), diabetes, smoking, coronary heart disease, and valvular heart disease (**Fig. 1**). The data on modifiable risk factors are briefly reviewed.

## Hypertension

Elevated blood pressure is highly predictive of risk of AF.[25,42,43] In the FHS, hypertension was associated with 40% and 50% increased risk of AF in woman and men,[43] respectively. Elevated systolic pressure, diastolic pressure, and pulse pressure have been shown highly predictive of AF risk.[25,44] Even systolic blood pressure that approaches the upper limit of normal is predictive of incident AF in healthy middle-aged men.[42] Data from the biracial ARIC study confirm that the attributable risk of elevated blood pressure for incident AF, 21.6%, was the highest of the modifiable risk factors.[45]

Hypertension is strongly associated with HF.[46–48] In the FHS, hypertension was associated with a 3-fold and 2-fold risk of HF in women and men, respectively, and 59% of cases in women and 39% of cases in men were attributable to hypertension.[48] In adults over 65 years, elevated pulse pressure is more predictive of HF than systolic pressure.[46]

## Obesity

Studies have demonstrated an independent association of elevated BMI and risk of AF.[49–52] A meta-analysis of 5 population-based cohorts found that obesity (BMI $\geq$30 kg/m$^2$) is associated with a 49% increased risk of AF.[53] A dose-response relationship exits such that an increase in BMI by 1 unit increases AF risk by 3% to 4.7%. Because of the obesity epidemic, the attributable risk of BMI for AF has increased over the past 5 decades.[7]

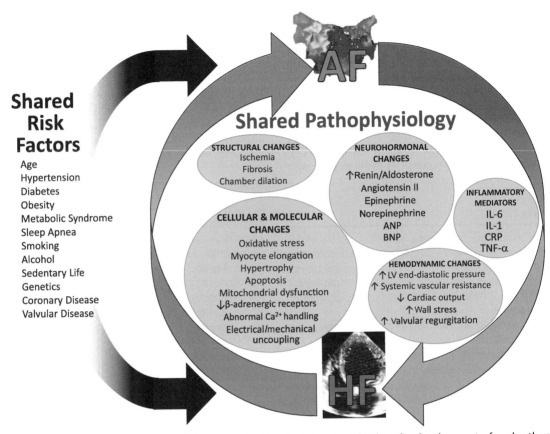

**Fig. 1.** AF and HF share common risk factors and pathophysiology that lead to the development of each other
CO, cardiac output; CRP, C reactive protein; IL, interleukin; LVEDP, left ventricular end diastolic volume; SVR, sys
temic vascular resistance; TNF, tumor necrosis factor.

Elevated BMI has been associated with risk of HF. In the FHS, after adjusting for HF risk factors, women with obesity were found to have greater than 2-fold risk of HF. Obesity in men was associated with a 90% increased risk of HF. A similar dose response was observed such that an increase in BMI by 1 unit the risk of HF increased by 7% in women and 5% in men.[54]

### Obstructive Sleep Apnea

OSA is highly prevalent and is strongly associated with risk of AF.[50,55] Sleep-disordered breathing was associated with a 4-fold risk of AF in the Sleep Heart Health Study.[55] In the Olmsted cohort, OSA was highly predictive of AF within 5 years of its diagnosis.[50] OSA also is associated with 2-fold risk of postoperative AF,[56] and recurrent AF after cardioversion[57] and ablation.[58]

OSA is associated with risk of HF.[59,60] Sleeping-disordered breathing was found in 37% of patients with HF undergoing polysomnography.[60] In the Sleep Heart Health Study, a dose-response was found, in those with apnea-hypopnea index

greater than 11, a 2.3 relative risk increase of prevalent HF was observed.[59]

### Diabetes

A meta-analysis of cohort studies reported that the relative risk for AF of prediabetes was approxi mately 1.2 and for diabetes was approximately 1.3.[61] Longer duration of AF and worse glycemic control have been associated with AF. The risk o AF increases by 3% with each year of diabetes duration.[62] The attributable risk of diabetes has increased over the past 5 decades, mirroring trends in increased obesity and diabete prevalence.[7]

Diabetes is associated with increased risk o HF.[28,47,63] In the FHS, woman and men with diabetes were found to have 5-fold and 2-fol increased risk of HF, respectively.[63] In the Nationa Health and Nutrition Examination Surve (NHANES) study, an 85% increased incident H risk was observed in diabetics with similar risk i both men and women.[47] In older adults greate than or equal to 65 years, diabetes was associate with an approximately 3-fold risk of HF.[28]

## Smoking

A meta-analysis reported that both former (relative risk [RR] 1.09) and current (RR 1.33) smoking were associated with AF risk.[64] The meta-analysis confirmed a dose-response pattern with AF risk. The CHARGE-AF (Cohorts for Aging and Research in Genomic Epidemiology) also observed a 44% increased incidence of AF in individuals who reported current smoking.[25] Secondhand smoke exposure also has been associated with risk of AF.[65]

Tobacco smoking also has been associated with increased risk of HF.[47,66] The Health ABC study demonstrated a dose-response pattern on HF risk.[67] The NHANES study showed a 49% increased risk of HF associated with current smoking.[47] The findings were similar in the Coronary Artery Surgery Study, which showed a 47% increased risk of HF.[68] In the NHANES study, the population attributed risk of smoking was only second to coronary heart disease for the development of HF.

## BIDIRECTIONAL ASSOCIATION OF ATRIAL FIBRILLATION AND HEART FAILURE

AF is a common comorbidity in patients with HFpEF, with prevalence ranging from 25% to 39% in clinical trials[69,70] and population-based,[30,71] registry,[23] and hospitalized cohorts.[72,73] In patients with HFrEF the prevalence of AF increases with worsening New York Heart Association class, ranging from 4.2% for class I to 49.8% for class IV.[74] Population-based studies have reported that HF confers a 2-fold to 4-fold risk of developing AF in blacks and whites.[25,75] A similar increased risk of AF is observed in patients with HFpEF, and this risk increased with worsening grade of diastolic dysfunction.[76]

Conversely, a meta-analysis showed that patients with AF have a 5-fold increased risk of HF.[6] Although several population-based cohort studies have shown that AF increases the risk of HF[27,77–79] and vice versa,[40,41,80] the temporality is harder to establish, in part because AF is sometimes unrecognized or undiagnosed.[81] In the CHS, 10% of participants developed AF and antecedent HF was associated with 2-fold increased risk AF whereas 32% of participants developed HF and antecedent AF was associated with an approximately 2-fold risk of HF.[82] The FHS assessed the temporal association and reported that among individuals with both conditions, 41% had HF first, 38% had AF first, and 21% had both diagnosed on the same day.[83] A subsequent study showed a trend toward prevalent AF more strongly associated with incident HFpEF than HFrEF (hazard ratio of 2.34 vs 1.32).[84] In the Olmsted County cohort, of

those with AF who developed incident HF, 61% had HFpEF and 39% had HFrEF.[85] HFpEF in patients with AF also may be underappreciated. In a study of patients with HFpEF undergoing ablation for paroxysmal AF, 25% of patients were found to have early signs of HF that was only clinically evident with invasive measure of left atrial pressure during exercise with arm ergometry.[86]

The strong association of AF and HF observed in population studies have been supported by basic and translational studies showing shared pathophysiology, including neurohormonal and proinflammatory activation and mechanoelectrical remodeling (see **Fig. 1**).[87–90]

## IMPACT OF ATRIAL FIBRILLATION AND HEART FAILURE ON MORTALITY

AF is associated with increased risk of death, and there is a gender interaction: in the FHS, the odds of death in women and men are 1.9 and 1.5, respectively. A meta-analysis confirmed the higher risk of death in women compared with men (RR 1.12).[91] At 10-year follow-up of women and men ages 55 years to 74 years, only 42.4% and 38.5%, respectively, with AF were surviving compared with 79.1% and 70% of women and men without AF. In Medicare beneficiaries older than 65 years, death was the most frequent outcome in individuals with AF and 5 years after developing AF, the death rate approached 50%.[92] Even in those without cardiovascular or valvular disease, AF is associated with 2-fold risk of death.[5] Excess mortality appears early after initial diagnosis of AF.[5] Although more recent data show that death attributable to AF may be declining over time,[7,23] perhaps owing to improved detection and treatment, AF continues to lend substantial risk of death particular in those with HF (both systolic and diastolic),[80,83,93,94] myocardial infarction,[95,96] coronary artery bypass surgery,[97,98] and stroke.[99]

The impact of AF and HF on mortality differs according to temporal onset of AF and is greatest when AF occurs in patients with preexisting HF. The FHS showed that in participants with antecedent AF or HF, the subsequent development of the other disease was associated with increased mortality. Preexisting HF negatively affected survival in individuals with AF, but preexisting AF did not have an impact on survival in those with HF.[83] In a more contemporary FHS sample (1980–2012), the presence of both AF and HF was found to confer a higher mortality risk compared with those without the other condition.[84] The incidence rates of death (per 1000 patient-years) of participants with new AF and prevalent HFpEF or HFrEF were

257 and 302 compared with 120 in those without HF. This risk was greater in those with HFrEF and AF (HR 2.72). The incidence rate of death (per 1000 patient-years) in participants with new HF and prevalent AF was 290 compared with 244 without AF (**Fig. 2**). Similarly, in the Olmsted County cohort, those with prevalent AF and new HF had a 29% increased risk of death, whereas those with prevalent HF and new AF had more than 2-fold increased risk of death.[100] When AF developed greater than 1-year after the diagnosis of HF the risk of death was 3-fold. The PRESERVE study also reported that incident AF was associated with a higher risk of death (HR 1.67) compared with prevalent AF (HR 1.13).[70] In a UK registry study, incident AF, HF, or both caused significantly worse mortality than those with the condition at baseline.[101] A meta-analysis of 33 observational studies found incident AF associated with increased mortality in both HFpEF and HFrEF. The relative risk of mortality did not differ between paroxysmal and persistent AF.[102] The difference in survival between prevalent and incident AF may due to those with prevalent AF, representing a pre-selected survivor group in which adaptations occur over time prior to HF incidence, whereas those with incident AF have less time for adaptation.[103] Meta-analysis of randomized controlled trials and observational studies show that AF is associated with higher mortality in HFpEF[93,94] than HFrEF,[94] although the association was weak (HR range 1.17–1.40). Whether AF directly contributes to enhanced mortality or merely serves as a marker for more advanced HF is uncertain.[104]

Clinical drug trials also have shown that AF is not only associated with adverse cardiovascular events

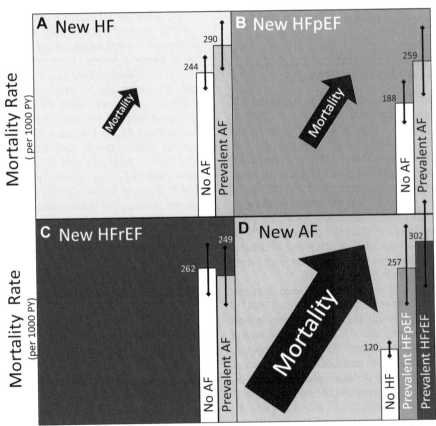

**Fig. 2.** Comparison of death rates in individuals with AF and HF by prevalence of the other condition. (*A*). Death rate of individuals with prevalent AF who subsequently develop HF compared with those without AF who develop HF. (*B*). Death rate of individuals with prevalent AF who subsequently develop HFpEF compared with those without AF who develop HFpEF. (*C*). Death rate of individuals with prevalent AF who subsequently develop HFrEF compared with those without AF who develop HFrEF. (*D*). Death rate of individuals with prevalent HFpEF or HFrEF who subsequently develop AF compared with those without HF who develop AF. Mortality is significantly increased in HF individuals who develop AF compared with AF individuals who develop HF highlighting importance of prevention and treatment of AF in HF patients. (*From* Wang TJ, Larson MG, Levy D, et al. Temporal relations of atrial fibrillation and congestive heart failure and their joint influence on mortality: the Framingham Heart Study. Circulation 2003;107(23):2923; with permission.)

(HF hospitalization and stroke) in HFpEF[105,106] and HFrEF[105] but also with increased mortality in HFpEF and HFrEF.[107] The impact of AF on adverse effects on HFpEF may be more in women.[106] In the BEST (Beta-Blocker Evaluation in Survival Trial) trial, patients with HFrEF and incident AF had 2-fold risk of mortality and 4.5-fold risk of HF hospitalization compared with those without AF.[108] In a post hoc analysis of the PARADIGM-HF and ATMOSPHERE HF trials, patients with paroxysmal AF had a higher risk of the primary composite endpoint of cardiovascular death or hospitalization, HF hospitalization, or stroke compared with those who did not have AF.[109]

The FHS showed that although prevalent AF is more strongly associated with incident HFpEF than HFrEF, those with new HFrEF had higher mortality compared with those with new HFpEF.[84] Data from registry studies are mixed. A study of Medicare claims for 66,357 hospitalized patients with AF and HF found that AF was associated with higher 30-day mortality only in those with HFpEF.[110] In the Swedish Heart Failure Registry, AF was associated with an equally increased risk of death, HF hospitalization, and stroke/transient ischemic attack irrespective of ejection fraction.[111] Similarly, in a large retrospective cohort study of 7156 patients with AF and HF, there was no difference in stroke or all-cause mortality if patients were stratified by EF.[112] Short-term mortality may be higher, however, in patients with AF and HFpEF after hospitalization. Results from meta-analysis are equally mixed, with one showing higher mortality with HFpEF,[93] another with HFrEF,[113] and a third showed similar mortality in both subtypes of HF.[94]

## SUMMARY

AF and HF are global epidemics that share common risk factors and have complex interactions. The prevalence of both AF and HF is increasing. There are important differences in AF and HF risk based on gender and race. AA individuals, despite having a lower lifetime risk of AF and HF, have worse outcomes. In addition, they are more likely than whites to develop HF. The existence of both AF and HF has substantial and additive impacts on mortality and cardiovascular morbidity. Improved preventive and treatment strategies for AF and HF are necessary to mitigate the morbidity, mortality, and economic burden of this double-edged sword.

## REFERENCES

1. Chugh SS, Havmoeller R, Narayanan K, et al. Worldwide epidemiology of atrial fibrillation: a global burden of disease 2010 study. Circulation 2014;129(8):837–47.

2. Colilla S, Crow A, Petkun W, et al. Estimates of current and future incidence and prevalence of atrial fibrillation in the U.S. adult population. Am J Cardiol 2013;112(8):1142–7.

3. Ruddox V, Sandven I, Munkhaugen J, et al. Atrial fibrillation and the risk for myocardial infarction, all-cause mortality and heart failure: a systematic review and meta-analysis. Eur J Prev Cardiol 2017;24(14):1555–66.

4. Santangeli P, Di Biase L, Bai R, et al. Atrial fibrillation and the risk of incident dementia: a meta-analysis. Heart Rhythm 2012;9(11):1761–8.

5. Benjamin EJ, Wolf PA, D'Agostino RB, et al. Impact of atrial fibrillation on the risk of death: the Framingham Heart Study. Circulation 1998;98(10):946–52.

6. Odutayo A, Wong CX, Hsiao AJ, et al. Atrial fibrillation and risks of cardiovascular disease, renal disease, and death: systematic review and meta-analysis. BMJ 2016;354:i4482.

7. Schnabel RB, Yin X, Gona P, et al. 50 year trends in atrial fibrillation prevalence, incidence, risk factors, and mortality in the Framingham Heart Study: a cohort study. Lancet 2015;386(9989):154–62.

8. Patel NJ, Deshmukh A, Pant S, et al. Contemporary trends of hospitalization for atrial fibrillation in the United States, 2000 through 2010: implications for healthcare planning. Circulation 2014;129(23):2371–9.

9. Kim MH, Johnston SS, Chu BC, et al. Estimation of total incremental health care costs in patients with atrial fibrillation in the United States. Circ Cardiovasc Qual Outcomes 2011;4(3):313–20.

10. Benjamin EJ, Virani SS, Callaway CW, et al. Heart disease and stroke statistics-2018 update: a report from the American Heart Association. Circulation 2018;137(12):e67–492.

11. Heidenreich PA, Albert NM, Allen LA, et al. Forecasting the impact of heart failure in the United States: a policy statement from the American Heart Association. Circ Heart Fail 2013;6(3):606–19.

12. Weng LC, Preis SR, Hulme OL, et al. Genetic predisposition, clinical risk factor burden, and lifetime risk of atrial fibrillation. Circulation 2018;137(10):1027–38.

13. Mou L, Norby FL, Chen LY, et al. Lifetime risk of atrial fibrillation by race and socioeconomic status: ARIC study (atherosclerosis risk in communities). Circ Arrhythm Electrophysiol 2018;11(7):e006350.

14. Magnussen C, Niiranen TJ, Ojeda FM, et al. Sex differences and similarities in atrial fibrillation epidemiology, risk factors, and mortality in community cohorts: results from the BiomarCaRE consortium (biomarker for cardiovascular risk assessment in Europe). Circulation 2017;136(17):1588–97.

15. Staerk L, Wang B, Preis SR, et al. Lifetime risk of atrial fibrillation according to optimal, borderline, or elevated levels of risk factors: cohort study

based on longitudinal data from the Framingham Heart Study. BMJ 2018;361:k1453.

16. Lloyd-Jones DM, Larson MG, Leip EP, et al. Lifetime risk for developing congestive heart failure: the Framingham Heart Study. Circulation 2002; 106(24):3068–72.

17. Bleumink GS, Knetsch AM, Sturkenboom MC, et al. Quantifying the heart failure epidemic: prevalence, incidence rate, lifetime risk and prognosis of heart failure the Rotterdam Study. Eur Heart J 2004; 25(18):1614–9.

18. Huffman MD, Berry JD, Ning H, et al. Lifetime risk for heart failure among white and black Americans: cardiovascular lifetime risk pooling project. J Am Coll Cardiol 2013;61(14):1510–7.

19. Rodriguez CJ, Soliman EZ, Alonso A, et al. Atrial fibrillation incidence and risk factors in relation to race-ethnicity and the population attributable fraction of atrial fibrillation risk factors: the Multi-Ethnic Study of Atherosclerosis. Ann Epidemiol 2015;25(2):71–6, 76.e1.

20. Ko D, Rahman F, Schnabel RB, et al. Atrial fibrillation in women: epidemiology, pathophysiology, presentation, and prognosis. Nat Rev Cardiol 2016;13(6):321–32.

21. Staerk L, Sherer JA, Ko D, et al. Atrial fibrillation: epidemiology, pathophysiology, and clinical outcomes. Circ Res 2017;120(9):1501–17.

22. Heeringa J, van der Kuip DA, Hofman A, et al. Prevalence, incidence and lifetime risk of atrial fibrillation: the Rotterdam study. Eur Heart J 2006; 27(8):949–53.

23. Piccini JP, Hammill BG, Sinner MF, et al. Incidence and prevalence of atrial fibrillation and associated mortality among Medicare beneficiaries, 1993-2007. Circ Cardiovasc Qual Outcomes 2012;5(1): 85–93.

24. Murphy NF, Simpson CR, Jhund PS, et al. A national survey of the prevalence, incidence, primary care burden and treatment of atrial fibrillation in Scotland. Heart 2007;93(5):606–12.

25. Alonso A, Krijthe BP, Aspelund T, et al. Simple risk model predicts incidence of atrial fibrillation in a racially and geographically diverse population: the CHARGE-AF consortium. J Am Heart Assoc 2013;2(2):e000102.

26. Levy D, Kenchaiah S, Larson MG, et al. Long-term trends in the incidence of and survival with heart failure. N Engl J Med 2002;347(18):1397–402.

27. Gottdiener JS, Arnold AM, Aurigemma GP, et al. Predictors of congestive heart failure in the elderly: the Cardiovascular Health Study. J Am Coll Cardiol 2000;35(6):1628–37.

28. Chen YT, Vaccarino V, Williams CS, et al. Risk factors for heart failure in the elderly: a prospective community-based study. Am J Med 1999;106(6): 605–12.

29. Redfield MM, Jacobsen SJ, Burnett JC Jr, et al. Burden of systolic and diastolic ventricular dysfunction in the community: appreciating the scope of the heart failure epidemic. JAMA 2003; 289(2):194–202.

30. Vasan RS, Larson MG, Benjamin EJ, et al. Congestive heart failure in subjects with normal versus reduced left ventricular ejection fraction: prevalence and mortality in a population-based cohort. J Am Coll Cardiol 1999;33(7):1948–55.

31. Dewland TA, Olgin JE, Vittinghoff E, et al. Incident atrial fibrillation among Asians, Hispanics, blacks, and whites. Circulation 2013;128(23):2470–7.

32. Go AS, Hylek EM, Phillips KA, et al. Prevalence of diagnosed atrial fibrillation in adults: national implications for rhythm management and stroke prevention: the AnTicoagulation and Risk Factors in Atrial Fibrillation (ATRIA) Study. JAMA 2001;285(18): 2370–5.

33. Alonso A, Agarwal SK, Soliman EZ, et al. Incidence of atrial fibrillation in whites and African-Americans: the atherosclerosis risk in communities (ARIC) study. Am Heart J 2009;158(1):111–7.

34. Benjamin EJ, Blaha MJ, Chiuve SE, et al. Heart disease and stroke statistics-2017 update: a report from the American Heart Association. Circulation 2017;135(10):e146–603.

35. Marcus GM, Alonso A, Peralta CA, et al. European ancestry as a risk factor for atrial fibrillation in African Americans. Circulation 2010;122(20):2009–15.

36. Magnani JW, Norby FL, Agarwal SK, et al. Racial differences in atrial fibrillation-related cardiovascular disease and mortality: the Atherosclerosis Risk in Communities (ARIC) Study. JAMA Cardiol 2016;1(4):433–41.

37. Bahrami H, Kronmal R, Bluemke DA, et al. Differences in the incidence of congestive heart failure by ethnicity: the multi-ethnic study of atherosclerosis. Arch Intern Med 2008;168(19):2138–45.

38. Kalogeropoulos A, Georgiopoulou V, Kritchevsky SB, et al. Epidemiology of incident heart failure in a contemporary elderly cohort: the health, aging, and body composition study. Arch Intern Med 2009; 169(7):708–15.

39. Bibbins-Domingo K, Pletcher MJ, Lin F, et al. Racial differences in incident heart failure among young adults. N Engl J Med 2009;360(12):1179–90.

40. Benjamin EJ, Levy D, Vaziri SM, et al. Independent risk factors for atrial fibrillation in a population based cohort. The Framingham Heart Study. JAMA 1994;271(11):840–4.

41. Lloyd-Jones DM, Wang TJ, Leip EP, et al. Lifetime risk for development of atrial fibrillation: the Framingham Heart Study. Circulation 2004;110(9): 1042–6.

42. Grundvold I, Skretteberg PT, Liestol K, et al. Upper normal blood pressures predict incident atrial

fibrillation in healthy middle-aged men: a 35-year follow-up study. Hypertension 2012;59(2):198–204.

43. Kannel WB, Wolf PA, Benjamin EJ, et al. Prevalence, incidence, prognosis, and predisposing conditions for atrial fibrillation: population-based estimates. Am J Cardiol 1998;82(8A):2N–9N.

44. Mitchell GF, Vasan RS, Keyes MJ, et al. Pulse pressure and risk of new-onset atrial fibrillation. JAMA 2007;297(7):709–15.

45. Huxley RR, Lopez FL, Folsom AR, et al. Absolute and attributable risks of atrial fibrillation in relation to optimal and borderline risk factors: the Atherosclerosis Risk in Communities (ARIC) study. Circulation 2011;123(14):1501–8.

46. Chae CU, Pfeffer MA, Glynn RJ, et al. Increased pulse pressure and risk of heart failure in the elderly. JAMA 1999;281(7):634–9.

47. He J, Ogden LG, Bazzano LA, et al. Risk factors for congestive heart failure in US men and women: NHANES I epidemiologic follow-up study. Arch Intern Med 2001;161(7):996–1002.

48. Levy D, Larson MG, Vasan RS, et al. The progression from hypertension to congestive heart failure. JAMA 1996;275(20):1557–62.

49. Frost L, Hune LJ, Vestergaard P. Overweight and obesity as risk factors for atrial fibrillation or flutter: the Danish Diet, Cancer, and Health Study. Am J Med 2005;118(5):489–95.

50. Gami AS, Hodge DO, Herges RM, et al. Obstructive sleep apnea, obesity, and the risk of incident atrial fibrillation. J Am Coll Cardiol 2007;49(5):565–71.

51. Murphy NF, MacIntyre K, Stewart S, et al. Long-term cardiovascular consequences of obesity: 20-year follow-up of more than 15 000 middle-aged men and women (the Renfrew-Paisley study). Eur Heart J 2006;27(1):96–106.

52. Wang TJ, Parise H, Levy D, et al. Obesity and the risk of new-onset atrial fibrillation. JAMA 2004;292(20):2471–7.

53. Wanahita N, Messerli FH, Bangalore S, et al. Atrial fibrillation and obesity–results of a meta-analysis. Am Heart J 2008;155(2):310–5.

54. Kenchaiah S, Evans JC, Levy D, et al. Obesity and the risk of heart failure. N Engl J Med 2002;347(5):305–13.

55. Mehra R, Benjamin EJ, Shahar E, et al. Association of nocturnal arrhythmias with sleep-disordered breathing: the sleep heart health study. Am J Respir Crit Care Med 2006;173(8):910–6.

56. Qaddoura A, Kabali C, Drew D, et al. Obstructive sleep apnea as a predictor of atrial fibrillation after coronary artery bypass grafting: a systematic review and meta-analysis. Can J Cardiol 2014; 30(12):1516–22.

57. Kanagala R, Murali NS, Friedman PA, et al. Obstructive sleep apnea and the recurrence of atrial fibrillation. Circulation 2003;107(20):2589–94.

58. Ng CY, Liu T, Shehata M, et al. Meta-analysis of obstructive sleep apnea as predictor of atrial fibrillation recurrence after catheter ablation. Am J Cardiol 2011;108(1):47–51.

59. Shahar E, Whitney CW, Redline S, et al. Sleep-disordered breathing and cardiovascular disease: cross-sectional results of the Sleep Heart Health Study. Am J Respir Crit Care Med 2001;163(1):19–25.

60. Sin DD, Fitzgerald F, Parker JD, et al. Risk factors for central and obstructive sleep apnea in 450 men and women with congestive heart failure. Am J Respir Crit Care Med 1999;160(4):1101–6.

61. Aune D, Feng T, Schlesinger S, et al. Diabetes mellitus, blood glucose and the risk of atrial fibrillation: a systematic review and meta-analysis of cohort studies. J Diabetes Complications 2018;32(5):501–11.

62. Dublin S, Glazer NL, Smith NL, et al. Diabetes mellitus, glycemic control, and risk of atrial fibrillation. J Gen Intern Med 2010;25(8):853–8.

63. Kannel WB, Hjortland M, Castelli WP. Role of diabetes in congestive heart failure: the Framingham study. Am J Cardiol 1974;34(1):29–34.

64. Aune D, Schlesinger S, Norat T, et al. Tobacco smoking and the risk of atrial fibrillation: a systematic review and meta-analysis of prospective studies. Eur J Prev Cardiol 2018;25(13):1437–51.

65. Dixit S, Pletcher MJ, Vittinghoff E, et al. Second-hand smoke and atrial fibrillation: data from the health eHeart study. Heart Rhythm 2016;13(1):3–9.

66. Kannel WB, Belanger AJ. Epidemiology of heart failure. Am Heart J 1991;121(3 Pt 1):951–7.

67. Gopal DM, Kalogeropoulos AP, Georgiopoulou VV, et al. Cigarette smoking exposure and heart failure risk in older adults: the health, aging, and body composition study. Am Heart J 2012;164(2):236–42.

68. Hoffman RM, Psaty BM, Kronmal RA. Modifiable risk factors for incident heart failure in the coronary artery surgery study. Arch Intern Med 1994;154(4):417–23.

69. Linssen GC, Rienstra M, Jaarsma T, et al. Clinical and prognostic effects of atrial fibrillation in heart failure patients with reduced and preserved left ventricular ejection fraction. Eur J Heart Fail 2011;13(10):1111–20.

70. McManus DD, Hsu G, Sung SH, et al. Atrial fibrillation and outcomes in heart failure with preserved versus reduced left ventricular ejection fraction. J Am Heart Assoc 2013;2(1):e005694.

71. Bursi F, Weston SA, Redfield MM, et al. Systolic and diastolic heart failure in the community. JAMA 2006;296(18):2209–16.

72. Lenzen MJ, Scholte op Reimer WJ, Boersma E, et al. Differences between patients with a preserved and a depressed left ventricular function:

a report from the EuroHeart Failure Survey. Eur Heart J 2004;25(14):1214–20.

73. Masoudi FA, Havranek EP, Smith G, et al. Gender, age, and heart failure with preserved left ventricular systolic function. J Am Coll Cardiol 2003;41(2): 217–23.

74. Maisel WH, Stevenson LW. Atrial fibrillation in heart failure: epidemiology, pathophysiology, and rationale for therapy. Am J Cardiol 2003;91(6A):2D–8D.

75. Krahn AD, Manfreda J, Tate RB, et al. The natural history of atrial fibrillation: incidence, risk factors, and prognosis in the Manitoba Follow-Up Study. Am J Med 1995;98(5):476–84.

76. Tsang TS, Gersh BJ, Appleton CP, et al. Left ventricular diastolic dysfunction as a predictor of the first diagnosed nonvalvular atrial fibrillation in 840 elderly men and women. J Am Coll Cardiol 2002; 40(9):1636–44.

77. Andersson T, Magnuson A, Bryngelsson IL, et al. Gender-related differences in risk of cardiovascular morbidity and all-cause mortality in patients hospitalized with incident atrial fibrillation without concomitant diseases: a nationwide cohort study of 9519 patients. Int J Cardiol 2014;177(1):91–9.

78. Goyal A, Norton CR, Thomas TN, et al. Predictors of incident heart failure in a large insured population: a one million person-year follow-up study. Circ Heart Fail 2010;3(6):698–705.

79. Stewart S, Hart CL, Hole DJ, et al. A population-based study of the long-term risks associated with atrial fibrillation: 20-year follow-up of the Renfrew/Paisley study. Am J Med 2002;113(5):359–64.

80. Zakeri R, Chamberlain AM, Roger VL, et al. Temporal relationship and prognostic significance of atrial fibrillation in heart failure patients with preserved ejection fraction: a community-based study. Circulation 2013;128(10):1085–93.

81. Freedman B, Camm J, Calkins H, et al. Screening for atrial fibrillation: a report of the AF-SCREEN International Collaboration. Circulation 2017;135(19): 1851–67.

82. O'Neal WT, Qureshi W, Zhang ZM, et al. Bidirectional association between atrial fibrillation and congestive heart failure in the elderly. J Cardiovasc Med (Hagerstown) 2016;17(3):181–6.

83. Wang TJ, Larson MG, Levy D, et al. Temporal relations of atrial fibrillation and congestive heart failure and their joint influence on mortality: the Framingham Heart Study. Circulation 2003;107(23):2920–5.

84. Santhanakrishnan R, Wang N, Larson MG, et al. Atrial fibrillation begets heart failure and vice versa: temporal associations and differences in preserved versus reduced ejection fraction. Circulation 2016;133(5):484–92.

85. Chamberlain AM, Gersh BJ, Alonso A, et al. No decline in the risk of heart failure after incident atrial fibrillation: a community study assessing trends overall and by ejection fraction. Heart Rhythm 2017;14(6):791–8.

86. Meluzin J, Starek Z, Kulik T, et al. Prevalence and predictors of early heart failure with preserved ejection fraction in patients with paroxysmal atrial fibrillation. J Card Fail 2017;23(7):558–62.

87. Cha YM, Redfield MM, Shen WK, et al. Atrial fibrillation and ventricular dysfunction: a vicious electromechanical cycle. Circulation 2004;109(23):2839–43.

88. Li D, Fareh S, Leung TK, et al. Promotion of atrial fibrillation by heart failure in dogs: atrial remodeling of a different sort. Circulation 1999;100(1): 87–95.

89. Shinagawa K, Shi YF, Tardif JC, et al. Dynamic nature of atrial fibrillation substrate during development and reversal of heart failure in dogs. Circulation 2002;105(22):2672–8.

90. Shinbane JS, Wood MA, Jensen DN, et al. Tachycardia-induced cardiomyopathy: a review of animal models and clinical studies. J Am Coll Cardiol 1997;29(4):709–15.

91. Emdin CA, Wong CX, Hsiao AJ, et al. Atrial fibrillation as risk factor for cardiovascular disease and death in women compared with men: systematic review and meta-analysis of cohort studies. BMJ 2016;532:h7013.

92. Piccini JP, Hammill BG, Sinner MF, et al. Clinical course of atrial fibrillation in older adults: the importance of cardiovascular events beyond stroke. Eur Heart J 2014;35(4):250–6.

93. Cheng M, Lu X, Huang J, et al. The prognostic significance of atrial fibrillation in heart failure with a preserved and reduced left ventricular function: insights from a meta-analysis. Eur J Heart Fail 2014; 16(12):1317–22.

94. Mamas MA, Caldwell JC, Chacko S, et al. A meta-analysis of the prognostic significance of atrial fibrillation in chronic heart failure. Eur J Heart Fail 2009;11(7):676–83.

95. Jabre P, Jouven X, Adnet F, et al. Atrial fibrillation and death after myocardial infarction: a community study. Circulation 2011;123(19):2094–100.

96. Jabre P, Roger VL, Murad MH, et al. Mortality associated with atrial fibrillation in patients with myocardial infarction: a systematic review and meta-analysis. Circulation 2011;123(15): 1587–93.

97. Kaw R, Hernandez AV, Masood I, et al. Short- and long-term mortality associated with new-onset atrial fibrillation after coronary artery bypass grafting: a systematic review and meta-analysis. J Thorac Cardiovasc Surg 2011;141(5):1305–12.

98. Phan K, Ha HS, Phan S, et al. New-onset atrial fibrillation following coronary bypass surgery predicts long-term mortality: a systematic review and meta-analysis. Eur J Cardiothorac Surg 2015; 48(6):817–24.

99. Lin HJ, Wolf PA, Kelly-Hayes M, et al. Stroke severity in atrial fibrillation. The Framingham Study. Stroke 1996;27(10):1760–4.

100. Chamberlain AM, Redfield MM, Alonso A, et al. Atrial fibrillation and mortality in heart failure: a community study. Circ Heart Fail 2011;4(6):740–6.

101. Ziff OJ, Carter PR, McGowan J, et al. The interplay between atrial fibrillation and heart failure on long-term mortality and length of stay: insights from the, United Kingdom ACALM registry. Int J Cardiol 2018;252:117–21.

102. Odutayo A, Wong CX, Williams R, et al. Prognostic importance of atrial fibrillation timing and pattern in adults with congestive heart failure: a systematic review and meta-analysis. J Card Fail 2017;23(1):56–62.

103. Verma A, Kalman JM, Callans DJ. Treatment of patients with atrial fibrillation and heart failure with reduced ejection fraction. Circulation 2017; 135(16):1547–63.

104. Khan MA, Satchithananda DK, Mamas MA. The importance of interactions between atrial fibrillation and heart failure. Clin Med (Lond) 2016;16(3):272–6.

105. Olsson LG, Swedberg K, Ducharme A, et al. Atrial fibrillation and risk of clinical events in chronic heart failure with and without left ventricular systolic dysfunction: results from the Candesartan in Heart failure-Assessment of Reduction in Mortality and morbidity (CHARM) program. J Am Coll Cardiol 2006;47(10):1997–2004.

106. O'Neal WT, Sandesara P, Hammadah M, et al. Gender differences in the risk of adverse outcomes in patients with atrial fibrillation and heart failure with preserved ejection fraction. Am J Cardiol 2017;119(11):1785–90.

107. Dries DL, Exner DV, Gersh BJ, et al. Atrial fibrillation is associated with an increased risk for mortality and heart failure progression in patients with asymptomatic and symptomatic left ventricular systolic dysfunction: a retrospective analysis of the SOLVD trials. Studies of Left Ventricular Dysfunction. J Am Coll Cardiol 1998;32(3): 695–703.

108. Aleong RG, Sauer WH, Davis G, et al. New-onset atrial fibrillation predicts heart failure progression. Am J Med 2014;127(10):963–71.

109. Mogensen UM, Jhund PS, Abraham WT, et al. Type of atrial fibrillation and outcomes in patients with heart failure and reduced ejection fraction. J Am Coll Cardiol 2017;70(20):2490–500.

110. Eapen ZJ, Greiner MA, Fonarow GC, et al. Associations between atrial fibrillation and early outcomes of patients with heart failure and reduced or preserved ejection fraction. Am Heart J 2014;167(3): 369–75.e2.

111. Sartipy U, Dahlstrom U, Fu M, et al. Atrial fibrillation in heart failure with preserved, mid-range, and reduced ejection fraction. JACC Heart Fail 2017; 5(8):565–74.

112. Banerjee A, Taillandier S, Olesen JB, et al. Ejection fraction and outcomes in patients with atrial fibrillation and heart failure: the Loire Valley Atrial Fibrillation Project. Eur J Heart Fail 2012;14(3): 295–301.

113. Kotecha D, Chudasama R, Lane DA, et al. Atrial fibrillation and heart failure due to reduced versus preserved ejection fraction: a systematic review and meta-analysis of death and adverse outcomes. Int J Cardiol 2016;203:660–6.

# Pathophysiology of Atrial Fibrillation and Heart Failure: Dangerous Interactions

Hariharan Sugumar, MBBS[a,b,c,d],
Shane Nanayakkara, MBBS[a,b,e],
Sandeep Prabhu, MBBS, PhD[a,b,c,d],
Aleksandr Voskoboinik, MBBS[a,b,c,d],
David M. Kaye, MBBS, PhD[a,b,e],
Liang-Han Ling, MBBS, PhD[a,b,d],
Peter M. Kistler, MBBS, PhD[a,b,d],*

## KEYWORDS

- Atrial fibrillation • Heart failure • Pathophysiology • HFpEF • HFrEF • Cardiomyopathy
- Tachycardiomyopathy • Diastolic dysfunction

## KEY POINTS

- Combination of atrial fibrillation and heart failure (HFpEF and HFrEF) is strongly associated with increased mortality and morbidity.
- Atrial fibrillation can lead to or exacerbate HFrEF through tachycardia and irregularity.
- Atrial fibrillation can lead to or exacerbate HFpEF through loss of atrial systole, irregularity, and diffuse fibrosis.
- Heart failure maybe reversible or improve significantly with catheter ablation leading to the successful restoration of sinus rhythm.

## INTRODUCTION

Atrial fibrillation (AF) and heart failure (HF) frequently coexist and are associated with a significant increase in morbidity and mortality.[1] Nearly two-thirds of people with AF develop HF, whereas AF develops in one-third of people with preexisting HF.[1,2] There are pathologic mechanisms through which AF may contribute to HF and inversely how HF may precipitate AF.

Disclosure Statement: The authors have no conflicts of interest pertaining to this article. However, the following industry funding sources regarding activities outside the submitted work have been declared in accordance with ICMJE guidelines. P.M. Kistler has received funding from Abott for consultancy and speaking engagements. L.-H. Ling has received fellowship support from Medtronic, Biotronik, and Abott. H. Sugumar has received fellowship support from St Jude Medical and Medtronic. Additionally, these nonindustry funding sources are also disclosed: Drs H. Sugumar, S. Prabhu, L.-H. Ling, and A. Voskoboinik receive funding from Australian National Health and Medical Research Council and/or National Heart Foundation of Australia and/or Royal Australasian College of Physicians and/or Centre of Research Excellence in Cardiovascular Outcomes.

[a] Department of clinical research, The Baker Heart and Diabetes Institute, 75 Commercial road, Melbourne, Victoria, 3004 Australia; [b] Department of Cardiology, The Alfred Hospital, 55 Commercial road, Melbourne, Victoria, 3004, Australia; [c] Department of Cardiology, Royal Melbourne Hospital, 300 Grattan Street, Parkville, Victoria 3050, Australia; [d] Department of Medicine, University of Melbourne, Grattan Street, Parkville, Victoria, 3010, Australia; [e] Department of Medicine, Monash University, Victoria, 3800, Australia
* Corresponding author. Heart Centre, The Alfred Hospital, Commercial Road, Melbourne, Victoria 3004, Australia.
E-mail address: peter.kistler@baker.edu.au

More recently HF with preserved ejection fraction (HFpEF) has been recognized with a prevalence equivalent to HF with reduced ejection fraction (HFrEF).[1] AF seems more prevalent in HFpEF than in people with HFrEF.[1,3] This may in part be explained by AF being heavily weighted in the proposed diagnostic criteria[4] and that AF and HFpEF have an increasing prevalence in the older, overweight population.

### Heart Failure with Reduced Ejection Fraction

The contribution of arrhythmias to left ventricular (LV) systolic function was first described in 1913.[5] AF is the commonest cause of arrhythmia-induced cardiomyopathies.[5] AF-related HFrEF may be categorized as either type 1 or type 2.[5] Type 1 is AF/arrhythmia induced: AF is entirely responsible for systolic dysfunction, which normalizes on restoration of sinus rhythm. Type 2 is AF/arrhythmia mediated: AF exacerbates preexisting or underlying cardiomyopathy, which only partially recovers with restoration of sinus rhythm.

The recent CAMERA-MRI and CASTLE-AF trials included patients with type 1 and type 2 AF induced and mediated LV systolic dysfunction. They demonstrated an improvement or normalization of LV systolic function following restoration of sinus rhythm with catheter ablation.[6,7] These studies have challenged the dogma from earlier pharmacologic studies, which had concluded that rate and rhythm control strategies were equivalent.[8] Retrospective substudies had demonstrated a survival advantage in patients in sinus rhythm but this seemed to be offset by the toxicity of antiarrhythmic drugs and the discontinuation of anticoagulation.

### Heart Failure with Preserved Ejection Fraction

Similar to AF-HFrEF, AF and HFpEF commonly coexist.[1,9–11] There is a large overlap between AF and HFpEF but earlier studies have been inconsistent in the inclusion criteria because of lack of consensus on the definition of HFpEF.[12,13] It is still the early stages of understanding the physiologic impact and contribution of AF on HFpEF with recent studies revealing significantly reduced exercise capacity and cardiac output in people with AF-HFpEF.[9,10,14,15] The role of AF ablation and the effect on HFpEF in people with coexistent AF and HFpEF is the subject of current studies.

Despite the shared common risk factors, such as advancing age, hypertension, obstructive sleep apnea, obesity, and coronary artery disease, AF and HF exacerbate each other. This review provides an overview of the pathophysiologic relationship between AF and the two most common types of HF syndromes: HFrEF and HFpEF (**Fig. 1**). For the purpose of this review, these intertwined clinical entities are discussed in a structured manner. However, in reality, the interaction is more dynamic with these conditions exacerbating one another in a complex and interconnected manner.

### DEFINITIONS

The 2016 European Society of Cardiology HF guidelines provide the most recent update on the diagnosis of HF.[15] "Heart failure is defined as a clinical syndrome characterized by typical symptoms that may be accompanied by signs caused by structural and/or functional cardiac abnormality, resulting in a reduced cardiac output and/or

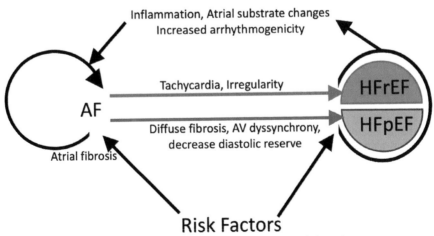

**Fig. 1.** Schematic representation of the pathophysiologic interaction between AF and HF. Common risk factors predispose to AF and HF including hypertension, advancing age, and obesity. AF and the HF subtypes can precipitate each other through complex physiologic effects. AV, atrioventricular.

elevated intracardiac pressure at rest or during stress."[15]

HFpEF is diagnosed when typical symptoms ± signs are accompanied by an LVEF greater than or equal to 50% plus elevated natriuretic peptides and evidence of diastolic dysfunction or relevant structural heart disease (LV hypertrophy or left atrial [LA] enlargement). The diagnosis of HFpEF in people with AF is more challenging.[14]

HFrEF is a simpler diagnosis with symptoms ± signs of HF and a LVEF less than 40%.

## ATRIAL FIBRILLATION CAUSING HEART FAILURE WITH REDUCED EJECTION FRACTION

AF contributes to HFrEF in one of two possible ways: tachycardia or irregularity.[5]

### Tachycardia

Whipple[16] was the first to describe experimental tachycardia-induced cardiomyopathy in 1962. This was confirmed in subsequent animal models of rapid ventricular pacing.[17] In canine and porcine models, Li and colleagues[18] and Tomita and colleagues[19] demonstrated that rapid ventricular pacing can induce HFrEF within weeks.[20] More importantly, this deterioration in LV function was largely reversible 1 to 2 weeks following normalization of heart rate.[17] The rate and duration of tachycardia are key factors in the time course and degree to which LV systolic dysfunction occurs.[17] This effect of tachycardia was present regardless of atrial or ventricular pacing.[17] Rapid ventricular pacing may result in systolic dysfunction not only through the effects of rate but also dyssynchrony.[5] Arrhythmia-mediated systolic dysfunction has four phases[21]:

- Early phase (3–7 days).
- Compensatory phase (>7 days): Normal systolic function.
- LV dysfunction phase (1–3 weeks): LV dilatation, systolic dysfunction, and neurohormonal activation.
- LV failure phase (>3 weeks): LV pump failure phase. LV dilatation with hemodynamic compromise.

In the early phase, there are adaptive changes with LV dilatation and a slight decline in LVEF but without compromise in cardiac output or systemic perfusion pressures. With sustained tachycardia LV dilatation and dysfunction occurs with a decline in myocardial contractile function.[22]

In parallel to the structural changes seen in tachycardia, there is an upregulation of neurohormonal signaling. Bioactive peptides, such as B-type natriuretic peptides (BNP), are increased in response to LV dilatation.[21,23,24] Given the lowered cardiac output, there is decreased renal blood flow to the distal tubules. As a compensatory evolutionary mechanism to maintain blood volume and perfusion, there is upregulation of renin-angiotensin-aldosterone system[25]; sympathetic activation; and upregulation of endothelin and inflammatory cytokines, such as tumor necrosis factor-α, which leads to a proinflammatory state and fluid accumulation. This continued fluid accumulation and proinflammatory response further exacerbate HF syndrome in addition to the effect of cardiomyocytes. There is hypertrophy of cardiomyocytes and reduction in cell division in animal models, which is likely to impact myocardial function.[21,26–28]

Tachycardia leads to changes in cellular calcium transport mechanisms. An increase in heart rate typically results in upregulation of $Ca^{2+}$ and the responsiveness of the myofilament to $Ca^{2+}$ with increased contractility; however, with sustained tachycardia, this relationship is downregulated.[29,30] Altered cellular $Ca^{2+}$ handling and defects in $Ca^{2+}$ cycling lead to a decrease in myocardial contractility[21,29,31,32] and ultimately cell death through apoptosis.[33]

As this progresses, in addition to the cellular changes, there is progressive alteration to the extracellular matrix (ECM) with loss of normal fibrillar collagen content and distribution and a decrease in the capacity of myocytes to bind to the ECM. Eventually, there is an increase in metalloproteinase activity leading to loss of ECM.[34,35] The LV dilatation that occurs is associated with lengthening of existing myocytes rather than an increase in cross-sectional area.[35]

This combination of altered cellular $Ca^{2+}$ handling, increased apoptosis, myocyte lengthening, inflammation, LV dilatation, and alteration to ECM leads to progressive LV dysfunction.

### Irregularity

Data is limited on the pathophysiologic and cellular effects of irregular ventricular contraction seen in those with rate-controlled AF. Intracellular calcium handling is a critical part of myocyte function. Animal studies have demonstrated that irregular contraction results in reduced expression of sarcoplasmic reticulum calcium ATPase and reduction in peak calcium transients with a corresponding reduction in ATPase protein expression signaling the adverse myocardial cellular effects of irregularity.[36] The contribution of irregularity in the presence of adequate rate control had been underappreciated and may be associated with significant hemodynamic consequences.[37,38] Normalization of ejection fraction following intervention and regularization of rhythm in those with rate-controlled AF demonstrates the role and impact of irregularity in people with AF-HFrEF, which is otherwise unexplained.[6,37,39] The CAMERA MRI trial demonstrated significant improvements in HF symptoms, ejection fraction, and BNP in patients where sinus rhythm was restored with catheter ablation compared with rate-controlled AF.[6] Aside from AF, premature ventricular complex provide a clinical example of the impact irregularity may have on LV function.[38]

We are in the early stages of identifying genes that may contribute to the development of AF and/or HF. The relationship between the impact of AF, the adequacy of rate control, and the effect on the development of LV systolic dysfunction is highly variable.

In addition to the cellular effects of irregularity, genetic susceptibility could play an important role in determining the development of AF-related HFrEF.[5] More than 50 genetic mutations have been implicated involving encoding molecules responsible for cellular function, integrity, and/or cytoskeletal structure.[40,41] Currently, genetic mutations may be identified in only 30% of people with dilated cardiomyopathy. Four of the common mutations include titin (TTN), lamin A/C (LMNA), β-myosin heavy chain (MYH7), and cardiac troponin T (TNNT2) genes.[5,41] However, the genetic profile of AF-HFrEF subpopulation has not been reported previously and is the subject of current studies. There are reports of genes implicated in the development of familial AF that overlaps with dilated cardiomyopathy, such as 6q14-q16 and 10q22-q24.[42]

Randomized clinical trials in patients with systolic HF and AF that have incorporated catheter ablation have highlighted the improvements in LV systolic function, HF symptoms, and mortality reduction associated with the restoration of sinus rhythm[7,43] supporting the concept of AF-induced HFrEF.

## ATRIAL FIBRILLATION CAUSING HEART FAILURE WITH PRESERVED EJECTION FRACTION

AF potentiates the development and progression of HFpEF, with three key pathophysiologic processes:

1. Loss of atrial systole and irregularity
2. Tachycardia
3. Diffuse fibrosis

### Loss of Atrial Systole and Irregularity

Cardiac output and filling pressures are partly determined by LV filling during the diastolic phase.[44] Coordinated LA contraction has an important role to play in LV filling and cardiac output. The function of the left atrium during the diastolic phase is detailed:

- Isovolumetric relaxation: LA acts as a reservoir during isovolumetric relaxation.
- Rapid filling: There is rapid filling of the LV in early diastole following active relaxation of LV during which the LA acts as a conduit.
- Slow filling/diastasis. LV filling slows as LV pressure approaches LA pressure.
- Atrial systole. Atrial systole, in end diastole, is an active process. This is responsible for 30% of ventricular filling in subjects younger than 50 years old but up to 70% and more in people who are older.

As such, LA structure and function influences the diastolic LV filling and emptying, hence cardiac output.[45] Coordinated atrial contraction is estimated to contribute up to 20% of the cardiac output in sinus rhythm.[37,46,47] Loss of atrioventricular synchrony impairs diastolic filling, which in turn worsens diastolic function thereby leading to increased left-sided pressure and symptoms of HF.[48,49]

Irregularity in ventricular contraction seen in AF has been associated with reversible increased LA pressure.[37,50–52] This could be caused by decreased LV relaxation time because of shortened R-R intervals seen in AF and decreased LA emptying. The loss of atrial contraction results in incomplete LA emptying and elevation in LA pressure.[45] The increasing contribution of LA systole to LV filling with aging is an important mechanism in the increasing prevalence of AF and HFpEF in the older population.

### Tachycardia

Animal models evaluating ventricular effects of tachycardia are limited to tachycardia-induced cardiomyopathy. However, diastolic assessments following tachycardia in these models provide some insight into the diastolic effects.[19] Tomita and colleagues[19] used isovolumic pressure decline, chamber stiffness constant, myocardial stiffness constant, and peak early diastolic filling rate [peak (+)dD/dt] as parameters to determine the impact of tachycardia on diastolic function. There was initial LV hypertrophy with persistently prolonged isovolumic pressure decline and increased chamber stiffness constant and myocardial stiffness constant, which were consistent with persistently impaired diastolic function. The ventricular collagen fibril diameter seems to respond differently to sustained versus paroxysmal tachycardia. Sustained tachycardia was shown to decrease the fibril diameter compared with nonsustained tachycardia. Unlike the reversible nature of HFrEF with tachycardia, porcine animal model studies have demonstrated that sustained tachycardia for weeks led to impaired diastolic dysfunction, which did not recover.[35]

Furthermore, rapid ventricular rates shorten diastolic time, which results in decreased LA emptying and LV filling thereby reducing cardiac output and increasing LA pressure.

## Diffuse Fibrosis

Reactive interstitial fibrosis, infiltrative interstitial fibrosis, and replacement fibrosis are three types of ventricular fibrosis that have been described.[53] The interstitial fibrillar collagen network is important to the normal diastolic function of the ventricle.[53]

In animal and human studies of interstitial fibrosis in HFpEF, there is an increase in biomarkers of inflammation, such as C-reactive protein, soluble ST2, and tissue inhibitor of metalloproteinases-1.[54] Sympathetic and neurohormonal activation is thought to be responsible for increase in inflammation and diffuse fibrosis via increased collagen synthesis by myofibroblasts and decreased degradation through profibrotic signaling, such as soluble ST2 and tissue inhibitor of metalloproteinases-1.[53–55] This reactive interstitial fibrosis is at least partially reversible with specific therapies and intervention that interrupts the proinflammatory cycle.[43,53,56]

AF is associated with diffuse interstitial ventricular fibrosis as measured by T1 mapping on cardiac MRI.[57] With progression from paroxysmal to persistent AF, fibrosis increases significantly. Reversibility of interstitial fibrosis with restoration of sinus rhythm in people with AF-HFpEF is the subject of current studies.

Impaired diastolic reserve is defined as elevated filling pressure under stress, which is preserved during the resting state.[58] AF is likely to worsen diastolic reserve because of a combination of diffuse fibrosis, loss of atrial contribution to cardiac filling/output, irregularity, and tachycardia.

## HEART FAILURE CAUSING ATRIAL FIBRILLATION

There are multiple postulated mechanisms through which HF leads to AF. The effects of the failing LV may result in electrical, structural, and ionic atrial remodeling, which can facilitate and perpetuate AF.

### Neurohormonal Changes

HF results in a proinflammatory state, which is coupled with upregulation of the sympathetic system, the renin-angiotensin-aldosterone system, endothelin, and inflammatory cytokines with the final common pathway of structural remodeling mediated by diffuse fibrosis.[18] In animal models, the electrophysiologic consequence of interstitial fibrosis has been shown to include conduction slowing and heterogeneity.[18] Human atrial mapping studies performed in patients with HFrEF in sinus rhythm demonstrated a significant reduction in atrial voltage with conduction slowing and an increased susceptibility to AF.[59] Recently, BNP has been shown to modulate pulmonary vein arrhythmogenesis through altered calcium handling and favor the development of AF (see later).[60]

### Mechanoelectrical Effect and Changes to Conduction

In the failing heart LV filling pressures increase, which is then transferred to the left atrium. Chronic LA stretch portends anisotropy with increased dispersion of refractoriness and direct stimulation of stretch-activated channels leading to an increased vulnerability to AF.[48,61,62] Human studies of the atrial electroanatomic properties in HFrEF demonstrate prolongation in atrial refractoriness, conduction time, P wave duration, and an increase in fractionated electrograms compared with age-matched control subjects.[59]

### Ionic and Cellular Changes and Arrhythmogenesis

Significant changes to cardiac ion channels have been described in systolic HF. There is calcium overload and prolonged action potential because of decrease in $I_{to}$, $I_{Ca}$, and $I_{Ks}$ currents and an increase in the NCX current.[63,64] Furthermore, there is loss of atrial t-tubules, increased sarcoplasmic reticulum calcium content, and increased diastolic calcium leak as a result of increased atrial pressure.[65,66] HF, through elevated BNP levels and increased sarcoplasmic reticulum calcium content,[60] increases afterdepolarizations originating from the pulmonary veins recognized as the triggers for AF episodes.[63,64]

## SUMMARY

AF and HF are modern epidemics with significant morbidity and mortality. AF can cause HFrEF and

HFpEF through a range of pathophysiologic mechanisms including rapid ventricular rates, irregularity and loss of atrial systole. In turn, HF can lead to AF through elevated atrial pressure and activation of the sympathetic and renin-angiotensin systems. Reassuringly, randomized clinical trials demonstrate that the restoration of sinus rhythm with catheter ablation can arrest this dangerous interaction with significant improvements in symptoms and survival.

## REFERENCES

1. Santhanakrishnan R, Wang N, Larson MG, et al. Atrial fibrillation begets heart failure and vice versa: temporal associations and differences in preserved vs. reduced ejection fraction. Circulation 2016; 133(5):484–92.
2. Wang TJ, Larson MG, Levy D, et al. Temporal relations of atrial fibrillation and congestive heart failure and their joint influence on mortality: the Framingham Heart Study. Circulation 2003;107(23):2920–5.
3. Seiler J, Stevenson WG. Atrial fibrillation in congestive heart failure. Cardiol Rev 2010;18(1):38–50.
4. Reddy YNV, Carter RE, Obokata M, et al. A simple, evidence-based approach to help guide diagnosis of heart failure with preserved ejection fraction. Circulation 2018;138(9):861–70.
5. Sugumar H, Prabhu S, Voskoboinik A, et al. Arrhythmia induced cardiomyopathy. J Arrhythmia 2018;34(4):376–83.
6. Prabhu S, Taylor AJ, Costello BT, et al. Catheter ablation versus medical rate control in atrial fibrillation and systolic dysfunction (CAMERA-MRI). J Am Coll Cardiol 2017;70(16):1949–61.
7. Marrouche NF, Brachmann J, Andresen D, et al. Catheter ablation for atrial fibrillation with heart failure. N Engl J Med 2018;378(5):417–27.
8. Wyse DG, Waldo AL, DiMarco JP, et al. A comparison of rate control and rhythm control in patients with atrial fibrillation. N Engl J Med 2002; 347(23):1825–33.
9. Kaye DM, Silvestry FE, Gustafsson F, et al. Impact of atrial fibrillation on rest and exercise haemodynamics in heart failure with mid-range and preserved ejection fraction. Eur J Heart Fail 2017;19(12):1690–7.
10. Lam CS, Rienstra M, Tay WT, et al. Atrial fibrillation in heart failure with preserved ejection fraction: association with exercise capacity, left ventricular filling pressures, natriuretic peptides, and left atrial volume. JACC Heart Fail 2017;5(2):92–8.
11. Kotecha D, Lam CS, Van Veldhuisen DJ, et al. Heart failure with preserved ejection fraction and atrial fibrillation: vicious twins. J Am Coll Cardiol 2016; 68(20):2217–28.
12. Vaduganathan M, Michel A, Hall K, et al. Spectrum of epidemiological and clinical findings in patients with heart failure with preserved ejection fraction stratified by study design: a systematic review. Eur J Heart Fail 2016;18(1):54–65.
13. Patel RB, Vaduganathan M, Shah SJ, et al. Atrial fibrillation in heart failure with preserved ejection fraction: insights into mechanisms and therapeutics. Pharmacol Ther 2017;176:32–9.
14. Borlaug BA, Nishimura RA, Sorajja P, et al. Exercise hemodynamics enhance diagnosis of early heart failure with preserved ejection fraction. Circ Heart Fail 2010;3(5):588–95.
15. Ponikowski P, Voors AA, Anker SD, et al. 2016 ESC Guidelines for the diagnosis and treatment of acute and chronic heart failure: the Task Force for the diagnosis and treatment of acute and chronic heart failure of the European Society of Cardiology (ESC) developed with the special contribution of the Heart Failure Association (HFA) of the ESC. Eur Heart J 2016;37(27):2129–200.
16. Whipple GH. Reversible congestive heart failure due to chronic rapid stimulation of the normal heart. Proc N Engl Cardiovasc Soc 1962;20:39–40.
17. Shinbane JS, Wood MA, Jensen DN, et al. Tachycardia-induced cardiomyopathy: a review of animal models and clinical studies. J Am Coll Cardiol 1997;29(4):709–15.
18. Li D, Fareh S, Leung TK, et al. Promotion of atrial fibrillation by heart failure in dogs: atrial remodeling of a different sort. Circulation 1999;100(1): 87–95.
19. Tomita M, Spinale FG, Crawford FA, et al. Changes in left ventricular volume, mass, and function during the development and regression of supraventricular tachycardia-induced cardiomyopathy. Disparity between recovery of systolic versus diastolic function. Circulation 1991;83(2):635–44.
20. Byrne MJ, Raman JS, Alferness CA, et al. An ovine model of tachycardia-induced degenerative dilated cardiomyopathy and heart failure with prolonged onset. J Card Fail 2002;8(2):108–15.
21. Gopinathannair R, Etheridge SP, Marchlinski FE, et al. Arrhythmia-induced cardiomyopathies: mechanisms, recognition, and management. J Am Coll Cardiol 2015;66(15):1714–28.
22. Gopinathannair R, Sullivan R, Olshansky B. Tachycardia-mediated cardiomyopathy: recognition and management. Curr Heart Fail Rep 2009;6(4): 257–64.
23. Moe GW, Grima EA, Wong NL, et al. Dual natriuretic peptide system in experimental heart failure. J Am Coll Cardiol 1993;22(3):891–8.
24. Riegger GA, Elsner D, Kromer EP, et al. Atrial natriuretic peptide in congestive heart failure in the dog: plasma levels, cyclic guanosine monophosphate, ultrastructure of atrial myoendocrine cells and hemodynamic, hormonal, and renal effects. Circulation 1988;77(2):398–406.

25. Schrier RW, Abraham WT. Hormones and hemodynamics in heart failure. N Engl J Med 1999;341(8):577–85.

26. Spinale FG, de Gasparo M, Whitebread S, et al. Modulation of the renin-angiotensin pathway through enzyme inhibition and specific receptor blockade in pacing-induced heart failure: I. Effects on left ventricular performance and neurohormonal systems. Circulation 1997;96(7):2385–96.

27. Bradham WS, Bozkurt B, Gunasinghe H, et al. Tumor necrosis factor-alpha and myocardial remodeling in progression of heart failure: a current perspective. Cardiovasc Res 2002;53(4):822–30.

28. Lijnen P, Petrov V. Renin-angiotensin system, hypertrophy and gene expression in cardiac myocytes. J Mol Cell Cardiol 1999;31(5):949–70.

29. Cory CR, McCutcheon LJ, O'Grady M, et al. Compensatory downregulation of myocardial Ca channel in SR from dogs with heart failure. Am J Physiol 1993;264(3 Pt 2):H926–37.

30. Eising GP, Hammond HK, Helmer GA, et al. Force-frequency relations during heart failure in pigs. Am J Physiol 1994;267(6 Pt 2):H2516–22.

31. Mukherjee R, Hewett KW, Walker JD, et al. Changes in L-type calcium channel abundance and function during the transition to pacing-induced congestive heart failure. Cardiovasc Res 1998;37(2):432–44.

32. Perreault CL, Shannon RP, Komamura K, et al. Abnormalities in intracellular calcium regulation and contractile function in myocardium from dogs with pacing-induced heart failure. J Clin Invest 1992;89(3):932–8.

33. Kajstura J, Zhang X, Liu Y, et al. The cellular basis of pacing-induced dilated cardiomyopathy. Myocyte cell loss and myocyte cellular reactive hypertrophy. Circulation 1995;92(8):2306–17.

34. Spinale FG, Coker ML, Thomas CV, et al. Time-dependent changes in matrix metalloproteinase activity and expression during the progression of congestive heart failure: relation to ventricular and myocyte function. Circ Res 1998;82(4):482–95.

35. Spinale FG, Tomita M, Zellner JL, et al. Collagen remodeling and changes in LV function during development and recovery from supraventricular tachycardia. Am J Physiol 1991;261(2 Pt 2):H308–18.

36. Ling LH, Khammy O, Byrne M, et al. Irregular rhythm adversely influences calcium handling in ventricular myocardium: implications for the interaction between heart failure and atrial fibrillation. Circ Heart Fail 2012;5(6):786–93.

37. Clark DM, Plumb VJ, Epstein AE, et al. Hemodynamic effects of an irregular sequence of ventricular cycle lengths during atrial fibrillation. J Am Coll Cardiol 1997;30(4):1039–45.

38. Simantirakis EN, Prassopoulos VK, Chrysostomakis SI, et al. Effects of asynchronous ventricular activation on myocardial adrenergic innervation in patients with permanent dual-chamber pacemakers; an I(123)-metaiodobenzylguanidine cardiac scintigraphic study. Eur Heart J 2001;22(4):323–32.

39. Natale A, Zimerman L, Tomassoni G, et al. Impact on ventricular function and quality of life of transcatheter ablation of the atrioventricular junction in chronic atrial fibrillation with a normal ventricular response. Am J Cardiol 1996;78(12):1431–3.

40. Burke MA, Cook SA, Seidman JG, et al. Clinical and mechanistic insights into the genetics of cardiomyopathy. J Am Coll Cardiol 2016;68(25):2871–86.

41. Cahill TJ, Ashrafian H, Watkins H. Genetic cardiomyopathies causing heart failure. Circ Res 2013;113(6):660–75.

42. Lubitz SA, Yi BA, Ellinor PT. Genetics of atrial fibrillation. Heart Fail Clin 2010;6(2):239–47.

43. Prabhu S, Costello BT, Taylor AJ, et al. Regression of diffuse ventricular fibrosis following restoration of sinus rhythm with catheter ablation in patients with atrial fibrillation and systolic dysfunction: a substudy of the CAMERA MRI trial. JACC Clin Electrophysiol 2018;4(8):999–1007.

44. Cohen-Solal A. Left ventricular diastolic dysfunction: pathophysiology, diagnosis and treatment. Nephrol Dial Transplant 1998;13(Suppl 4):3–5.

45. Blume GG, McLeod CJ, Barnes ME, et al. Left atrial function: physiology, assessment, and clinical implications. Eur J Echocardiogr 2011;12(6):421–30.

46. Simantirakis EN, Koutalas EP, Vardas PE. Arrhythmia-induced cardiomyopathies: the riddle of the chicken and the egg still unanswered? Europace 2012;14(4):466–73.

47. Mukharji J, Rehr RB, Hastillo A, et al. Comparison of atrial contribution to cardiac hemodynamics in patients with normal and severely compromised cardiac function. Clin Cardiol 1990;13(9):639–43.

48. Cha YM, Redfield MM, Shen WK, et al. Atrial fibrillation and ventricular dysfunction: a vicious electromechanical cycle. Circulation 2004;109(23):2839–43.

49. Prabhu S, Voskoboinik A, Kaye DM, et al. Atrial fibrillation and heart failure: cause or effect? Heart Lung Circ 2017;26(9):967–74.

50. Wasmund SL, Li JM, Page RL, et al. Effect of atrial fibrillation and an irregular ventricular response on sympathetic nerve activity in human subjects. Circulation 2003;107(15):2011–5.

51. Daoud EG, Weiss R, Bahu M, et al. Effect of an irregular ventricular rhythm on cardiac output. Am J Cardiol 1996;78(12):1433–6.

52. Hauser J, Michel-Behnke I, Zervan K, et al. Noninvasive measurement of atrial contribution to the cardiac output in children and adolescents with congenital complete atrioventricular block treated with dual-chamber pacemakers. Am J Cardiol 2011;107(1):92–5.

53. Mewton N, Liu CY, Croisille P, et al. Assessment of myocardial fibrosis with cardiovascular magnetic resonance. J Am Coll Cardiol 2011;57(8):891–903.

54. Zile MR, Baicu CF, Ikonomidis JS, et al. Myocardial stiffness in patients with heart failure and a preserved ejection fraction. Circulation 2015;131(14): 1247–59.

55. Su MY, Lin LY, Tseng YH, et al. CMR-verified diffuse myocardial fibrosis is associated with diastolic dysfunction in HFpEF. JACC Cardiovasc Imaging 2014;7(10):991–7.

56. Diez J, Querejeta R, Lopez B, et al. Losartan-dependent regression of myocardial fibrosis is associated with reduction of left ventricular chamber stiffness in hypertensive patients. Circulation 2002;105(21): 2512–7.

57. Ling LH, Kistler PM, Ellims AH, et al. Diffuse ventricular fibrosis in atrial fibrillation: noninvasive evaluation and relationships with aging and systolic dysfunction. J Am Coll Cardiol 2012;60(23):2402–8.

58. Chattopadhyay S, Alamgir MF, Nikitin NP, et al. Lack of diastolic reserve in patients with heart failure and normal ejection fraction. Circ Heart Fail 2010;3(1): 35–43.

59. Sanders P, Morton JB, Davidson NC, et al. Electrical remodeling of the atria in congestive heart failure: electrophysiological and electroanatomic mapping in humans. Circulation 2003;108(12):1461–8.

60. Lin YK, Chen YC, Chen YA, et al. B-type natriuretic peptide modulates pulmonary vein arrhythmogenesis: a novel potential contributor to the genesis of atrial tachyarrhythmia in heart failure. J Cardiovasc Electrophysiol 2016;27(12):1462–71.

61. Solti F, Vecsey T, Kekesi V, et al. The effect of atrial dilatation on the genesis of atrial arrhythmias. Cardiovasc Res 1989;23(10):882–6.

62. Bode F, Katchman A, Woosley RL, et al. Gadolinium decreases stretch-induced vulnerability to atrial fibrillation. Circulation 2000;101(18):2200–5.

63. Staerk L, Sherer JA, Ko D, et al. Atrial fibrillation: epidemiology, pathophysiology, and clinical outcomes. Circ Res 2017;120(9):1501–17.

64. Li D, Melnyk P, Feng J, et al. Effects of experimental heart failure on atrial cellular and ionic electrophysiology. Circulation 2000;101(22):2631–8.

65. Eckstein J, Verheule S, de Groot NM, et al. Mechanisms of perpetuation of atrial fibrillation in chronically dilated atria. Prog Biophys Mol Biol 2008; 97(2–3):435–51.

66. Denham NC, Pearman CM, Caldwell JL, et al. Calcium in the pathophysiology of atrial fibrillation and heart failure. Front Physiol 2018;9:1380.

# Tackling Patient-Reported Outcomes in Atrial Fibrillation and Heart Failure
## Identifying Disease-Specific Symptoms?

Benjamin A. Steinberg, MD, MHS, FHRS[a,*],
Jonathan P. Piccini Sr, MD, MHS, FHRS[b,c]

**KEYWORDS**

- Atrial fibrillation • Heart failure • Patient-reported outcomes • Health-related quality of life

**KEY POINTS**

- Atrial fibrillation (AF) and heart failure (HF) each represent disease processes with significant impacts on health-related quality of life (hrQoL).
- hrQoL is best ascertained through the use of structured, well-validated patient-reported outcomes (PROs).
- Several PRO instruments have been developed and validated for measurement of disease-specific hrQoL domains in AF and HF.
- Some PRO instruments focus on overall AF disease-specific hrQoL, others on symptoms, and others on anticoagulation satisfaction.
- Interventions for AF and HF have demonstrated improvement in hrQoL, as measured by PROs.

Among patients with heart failure (HF), atrial fibrillation (AF) occurs in more than one-third, including up to half of those with severe HF.[1–3] Although both diseases are well known to significantly affect morbidity and mortality, they also account for high symptom burden and significantly impair health-related quality of life (hrQoL). Although improving quality of life remains a primary goal in the care of patients with AF and HF, measurement and improvement of hrQoL outcomes remains a major challenge. This review discusses the measurement of hrQoL in AF and HF, including its importance, tools for such measurement and discrimination, and implications for disease management to improve hrQoL in these high-risk patients.

## IMPORTANCE OF HEALTH-RELATED QUALITY OF LIFE

Separately, AF and HF each reduce hrQoL due to impaired functional status and high symptom

Disclosure Statement: Work reported in this publication was supported by the National Heart, Lung, and Blood Institute (United States) of the National Institutes of Health under Award Number K23HL143156 (to BAS). The content is solely the responsibility of the authors and does not necessarily represent the official views of the National Institutes of Health. The following relationships exist related to this presentation: B.A. Steinberg reports no other relevant relationships; J.P. Piccini receives funding for clinical research from Abbott (United States), ARCA biopharma, Boston Scientific (United States), Gilead (United States), Janssen Pharmaceuticals (United States), and NHLBI and serves as a consultant to Abbott, Allergan, ARCA Biopharma, Bayer, Biotronik, GSK, Johnson & Johnson, Medtronic, Motif Bio, Sanofi, and Phillips.
[a] Division of Cardiovascular Medicine, University of Utah Health Sciences Center, 30 North 1900 East, Room 4A100, Salt Lake City, UT 84132, USA; [b] Duke University Medical Center, Durham, NC, USA; [c] Duke Center for Atrial Fibrillation, Duke University Medical Center, Duke Clinical Research Institute, DUMC #3115, Durham, NC 27705, USA
* Corresponding author. Division of Cardiovascular Medicine, University of Utah Health Sciences Center, 30 North 1900 East, Room 4A100, Salt Lake City, UT 84132.
E-mail address: benjamin.steinberg@hsc.utah.edu

Cardiol Clin 37 (2019) 139–146
https://doi.org/10.1016/j.ccl.2019.01.013
0733-8651/19/© 2019 Elsevier Inc. All rights reserved.

burden. For patients with AF without HF, hrQoL has been found to be comparable with that of patients with an acute myocardial infarction.[4] Among patients with HF without AF, hrQoL is very poor for more than 20% of patients with HF and is associated with increased health care utilization, increased costs, and worse clinical prognosis.[5–7] These patients are less likely to report good outlook, more likely to be depressed, and subsequently limit their engagement in care.[8]

However, clinical outcomes among patients with concomitant HF and AF are dramatically worse than either disease alone,[3,9] and there is a reason to believe the impact on hrQoL is also compounded.[3] Patients with AF and congestive HF (CHF) in the Atrial Fibrillation and Congestive Heart Failure trial demonstrated Short Form 36 Physical Component Summary scores 1.3 standard deviations below the national average. Normal rhythm was associated with improved hrQoL, supporting some independent effects of AF, and the implementation of arrhythmia interventions for these patients (see later discussion).[10,11]

However, the routine and/or systematic measurement of hrQoL in clinical care of patients with AF and HF remains challenging, despite the availability of numerous tools to assess symptoms and hrQoL in these patients.

## MEASUREMENT OF HEALTH-RELATED QUALITY OF LIFE IN ATRIAL FIBRILLATION AND HEART FAILURE

Patient-reported outcomes (PROs) are best defined as "…any report of the status of a patient's health condition that comes directly from the patient…"[12]; they represent the most direct measurement of hrQoL, without influence of interpretation by the clinician or other health care personnel. The formal measurement of hrQoL can best be ascertained via structured, validated PROs. In addition, when performed using well-validated and well-calibrated tools, PROs can provide the well-controlled, quantitative evidence to support interventions to improve hrQoL. For each disease, AF and HF, several PRO tools have been developed to assess symptom

**Table 1**
**Summary of instruments for PRO measurement in AF and HF**

| PRO Tools | Structure | Sample Clinical Study Implementation |
|---|---|---|
| **AF** | | |
| AFEQT[14] | 4 Domains: (1) symptoms, (2) daily activities, (3) treatment concerns, (4) treatment satisfaction | ORBIT-AF registry,[57] CABANA trial[37] |
| AFSS[4] | 4 Domains: (1) AF burden, (2) global well-being, (3) AF symptom score, (4) health care utilization | RACE II trial,[58,59] CTAF trial[34] |
| AF-QoL[13] | 3 Domains: (1) psychological, (2) physical, (3) sexual | SARA trial[60] |
| MAFSI[16] | Single inventory of AF symptoms | CABANA trial[37] |
| SCL[61] | Single inventory of AF symptom frequency and severity | AFFIRM trial[17] |
| ASTA[62] | Single inventory of arrhythmia symptoms | SMURF study[63] |
| **HF** | | |
| KCCQ/ KCCQ-12[24,26] | 7 Domains: (1) physical limitation, (2) symptom frequency, (3) symptom severity, (4) symptom stability, (5) self-efficacy, (6) limitations to lifestyle, (7) quality of life; KCCQ-12 includes only #1,2,6,7 | STICH,[64] PARADIGM-HF,[44] TOPCAT[65] trials FDA cleared[25] |
| MLWHF | Cumulative Domains: HF symptoms, physical functioning, sleep, role function, sex, recreation, appetite, psychological/emotional, adverse effects of medication, hospitalization, medical costs | SOLVD,[66] A-HeFT[67] |
| CHQ | 3 Domains: (1) dyspnea, (2) fatigue, (3) emotional function | |

Patient-reported outcome tools developed specifically for HF and the symptoms they target.
*Abbreviations:* AFEQT, AF effect on quality of life; AF-QoL, AF quality of life scale; AFSS, University of Toronto AF severity scale; ASTA, Arrhythmia-Specific questionnaire in Tachycardia and Arrhythmia; CHQ, chronic heart failure questionnaire; KCCQ, Kansas City cardiomyopathy questionnaire; MAFSI, Mayo AF-specific symptom inventory; MLHF, Minnesota living with heart failure; SCL, symptom checklist.
*Adapted from* Mark DB. Assessing quality-of-life outcomes in cardiovascular clinical research. Nat Rev Cardio 2016;13:286–308; with permission.

status and hrQoL, some of which have been extensively validated and implemented (**Table 1**).

## Atrial Fibrillation Patient-Reported Outcomes

Care of patients with AF is multi-dimensional, including the treatment of comorbidities, management of symptoms, and prevention of sequelae, principally stroke. Therefore, AF-specific PROs may target different aspects of the disease, such as (1) overall health status and impact of the disease (eg, AF Effect on Quality of Life [AFEQT]); (2) detailed burden of specific, AF-related symptoms (eg, the symptom checklist, Mayo AF-specific Symptom Inventory [MAFSI]); and (3) the impact of oral anticoagulation on hrQoL (eg, Anticlot Treatment Survey). Because of the overlap of AF and HF symptoms, the present review focuses on the first 2 categories of AF-related PROs.

Several AF-specific PRO instruments have been developed, and they are validated to a varying degree. These PROs have been derived primarily to assess symptom burden in the setting of interventions, such as catheter ablation. Nevertheless, they have been deployed in a variety of clinical and research settings, to assess hrQoL in patients with AF.

Symptom checklists are a major component of AF PROs, and comprise at least a component of the 16-item AF Symptom Checklist (SCL) tool, the Toronto AF Symptom Severity Scale (AFSS), the MAFSI, and the AFEQT (**Box 1**).[13–18] Some are more closely tied to AF-specific symptoms than others and may include additional domains, such as psychological function or sexual activity, in addition to physical function or symptoms. For example, the MAFSI functions as a very specific symptom survey and includes the most common physical symptoms associated with AF, such as palpitations, dizziness, exertional intolerance, sense of low heart rate, and syncope or presyncope.[16] Others, such as AF-QoL, are structured more broadly across domains of Psychological, Physical, and Sexual Activity impacts, with many questions that are less specific for AF.[13] Because AF clearly affects hrQoL via multiple avenues (eg, symptoms, anxiety of disease, restriction of activity), different measurement tools for different interventions may be required to demonstrate impact across a variety of domains.

## Heart Failure Patient-Reported Outcomes

Similarly, PRO instruments have been developed to capture physical symptom burden, psychological and emotional domains, and overall quality of life among patients with HF. Furthermore, there is robust evidence supporting the use of HF PROs as intermediate endpoints via the FDA's Expedited

---

**Box 1**
**Potential atrial fibrillation–related symptoms included in the most common atrial fibrillation–specific PROs**

- Palpitations
- Irregular heart beat
- Pause in heart activity
- Sense of low heart rate
- Chest pain/pressure
- Lightheadedness/dizziness
- Flushing
- Swelling
- Syncope/Presyncope
- Anxiety about:
  - Impending episodes
  - AF-related sequelae
  - Procedures
  - Medication effects, including bleeding
  - Limitations of daily living
- Lack of appetite
- Difficulty with concentration
- Sleep disturbance
- Weakness
- Fatigue at rest
- Exercise intolerance
- Dyspnea at rest
- Dyspnea with exertion
- Treatment satisfaction
  - Control of AF
  - Relief of AF symptoms

---

Access for Premarket Approval pathway.[19] The most common HF PROs are summarized in **Table 1**, with the earliest being the Minnesota Living with Heart Failure questionnaire.[20–22] This 21-item instrument is summarized as a single score, without specifically targeted domains, and assesses the impact of HF on physical, emotional, social, and mental components of quality of life.[23]

The most well validated and the only HF PRO that is now qualified as a medical device development tool by the Food and Drug Administration is the Kansas City Cardiomyopathy Questionnaire (KCCQ).[24,25] The KCCQ includes PRO assessment of HF across 7 domains: Physical Limitation, Symptom Stability, Symptom Frequency, Symptom Burden, Self-Efficacy, Quality of Life, and Social Limitations. A shorter version, the KCCQ-12, has also been developed and validated to target specific domains, but maintain the reliability, responsiveness, and interpretability of the full-length version.[26] Therefore, the KCCQ-12 focuses primarily on domains most related to HF health status (physical limitation, symptom frequency, quality of life, and social limitation) and has been successfully deployed as a routine HF PRO measurement in busy clinical settings.[27] In clinical trials, the KCCQ has been found to be independently predictive of subsequent resource utilization and mortality among patients with HF.[5,7,28–30]

## DISEASE-SPECIFIC INTERVENTIONS AND OUTCOMES

### Improvement of Health-related Quality of Life in Atrial Fibrillation

In studies of AF interventions, PROs often track with clinical and arrhythmia outcomes. For example, in the AFFIRM study testing strategies of rate versus rhythm control, consistent maintenance of sinus rhythm was suboptimal, and clinical outcomes were not significantly different.[31] The PROs and hrQoL among a subset of patients in the 2 arms were not different.[17] Similarly, the CTAF trial tested several different antiarrhythmic drugs in rhythm control of AF[32]; there was improvement in hrQoL across agents tested, with some of the effect attenuated by recurrence of AF during follow-up.[33,34] In addition, there have been numerous studies comparing catheter ablation of AF to medical therapy (ie, antiarrhythmic drugs), which have demonstrated favorable results of ablation, with respect to maintaining sinus rhythm and hrQoL.[35,36] Furthermore, many of these studies have included much more aggressive monitoring for arrhythmia, and thus more detailed data on recurrence rates and AF burden. Contemporary data from the CABANA trial have also shown very favorable effects of catheter ablation on hrQoL in a broad population of patients with AF.[37] And in studies with longer follow-up, the effect of ablation on hrQoL seems sustained at 2 years, even among patients with recurrent AF.[16]

It is important to acknowledge that many studies used a variety of PROs, including both disease-specific as well as more generic hrQoL tools that operate independent of disease state. However, there is robust evidence in support of the specificity of disease-specific PROs, which may better discriminate improvement targeted at specific disease states and pathophysiology. In a study of 54 patients undergoing ablation, the 6-item AF6 questionnaire was found to be more responsive to hrQoL improvement following ablation, compared with the more generic, but longer, standard, SF-36 tool.[38]

### Improvement of Health-related Quality of Life in Heart Failure

Across HF studies, several successful interventions for morbidity and mortality have also been shown to improve PROs. In fact, the KCCQ has been found to reliably reflect clinical changes in HF status and statistically out-performed both the New York Heart Association (NYHA) classification and the 6-minute walk test.[39] Nonpharmacologic, noninvasive interventions, such as exercise training, have been shown to improve hrQoL among patients with HF.[40] And in the recent PARADIGM-HF study comparing sacubitril/valsartan versus enalapril, the KCCQ was collected in more than 90% of patients.[41] Sacubitril/valsartan was shown not only to improve clinical HF markers and mortality, but there was also substantial improvement in nearly all KCCQ physical and social activities. Even more aggressive and invasive HF treatments have also improved hrQoL—patients undergoing implantation of left-ventricular assist devices (LVADs) for end-stage HF again improved mortality, and demonstrated dramatic improvements in hrQoL, despite the morbidity of a major surgical procedure.[42]

### Interventions for Atrial Fibrillation and Heart Failure

However, most of these studies did not specifically target patients with concomitant AF and HF—prevalence of AF often hovered around one-third of those enrolled in major HF trials.[43–45] Given the unique risks and challenges of patients with concomitant AF and HF, several studies have specifically targeted these patients and have reported hrQoL outcomes.

The AF-CHF trial compared strategies of rate-only versus rhythm control among 1376 patients with AF and HF and found no differences in the rates of cardiovascular death (the primary endpoint).[46] And although hrQoL also did not differ between the 2 groups overall, maintenance of sinus rhythm was associated with improved NYHA class and hrQoL.[1] In fact, there is mounting evidence that targeted treatment of AF (ie, restoring and/or maintaining sinus rhythm) dramatically improves PROs among HF patients. Even short-term interventions, such as cardioversion, seem to improve exercise capacity for those who maintain sinus rhythm.[11]

More recently, trials of more definitive interventions for AF, in the setting of HF, have demonstrated favorable long-term results in this high-risk population. Several studies of catheter ablation, specifically in patients with AF and concomitant HF, have shown improvements in clinical outcomes.[47–49] In fact, the first

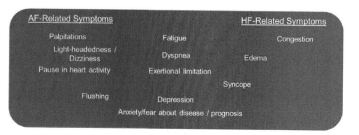

**Fig. 1.** Overlap in symptoms specific for AF versus HF.

study demonstrating a mortality benefit of ablation in AF, the CASTLE-AF trial, specifically targeted patients with AF and concomitant HF.[50] Subsequent meta-analyses of AF ablation in patients with HF (compared with medical therapy) have shown not only consistent clinical benefits, but also improvements in functional status and hrQoL.[51,52]

## DISCRIMINATING ATRIAL FIBRILLATION VERSUS HEART FAILURE HEALTH-RELATED QUALITY OF LIFE

A major unmet clinical challenge remains the discrimination of effects of AF versus HF in patients with both disease processes, with respect to both adverse clinical events and PROs. AF may manifest before or after the development of HF, and the temporal relationship may indicate distinct clinical phenotypes and subsequent outcomes. For example, the sequelae of persistent tachycardia, often due to AF, have been well described to lead to left-ventricular dysfunction and HF[53,54]; rhythm control interventions for AF in these specific patients seem to demonstrate significant benefits, compared with patients manifesting cardiomyopathy due to other causes.[55] Yet, AF may develop later in the HF process, and these patients likely represent different clinical phenotypes. Although there remains a role for rhythm control interventions such as ablation, clinical response is often more heterogeneous in this broader group of patients with HF.[48]

This variability in disease states limits our ability to identify the relative contributions of AF versus HF to poor hrQoL, across the population of patients with AF and HF. Disentangling the complex relationship between AF and HF is also limited by the significant overlap in symptomatology between the 2—each can account for relatively vague symptoms of dyspnea, exertional limitation, and fatigue, to name a few (**Fig. 1**). Therapeutic interventions specifically targeted to either AF or HF (as discussed earlier) may still provide mechanistic insight through understanding which patients are most likely to respond to specific interventions.

## PATIENT-REPORTED OUTCOMES AND CLINICIAN-REPORTED OUTCOMES

A major concern in the treatment of AF and HF symptoms is the distinction between PROs and clinician-reported outcomes (CROs). Several CROs are frequently used in these patients, such as the NYHA classification (for HF) and the European Heart Rhythm Association classification (for AF). These scales have been adopted and widely used as a way of classifying disease burden and/or functional status on a simple I–IV scale, as assessed and interpreted by the clinician. They frequently reflect the clinician's general impression of disease status or burden and provide little to no detail regarding the patient's experience and symptoms. Although there seems to be general concordance that higher worse status by CROs translates to higher symptom burden by PROs,[15,24] detailed, disease-specific PROs seem to be more sensitive and relevant outcomes for patients, particularly following interventions.[56] In both research and clinical settings, they can provide complementary information on individual patients and across patient cohorts.

## SUMMARY

hrQoL is best measured using disease-specific, validated PROs, and patients with AF and HF have significantly impaired hrQoL. Several well-designed and broadly implemented PRO instruments are available for both AF and HF and can easily measure hrQoL burden for each disease process. Disease-specific interventions for AF and HF, separately, have demonstrated improvements in both clinical outcomes and PROs, and emerging data support aggressive treatments for patients with both AF and HF. A better understanding of the diverse phenotypes of AF and HF, as well as the heterogeneous treatment effects of disease-specific interventions, is necessary to further disentangle the complex relationship between AF and HF.

## REFERENCES

1. Wang TJ, Larson MG, Levy D, et al. Temporal relations of atrial fibrillation and congestive heart

failure and their joint influence on mortality: the Framingham Heart Study. Circulation 2003;107: 2920–5.

2. Maisel WH, Stevenson LW. Atrial fibrillation in heart failure: epidemiology, pathophysiology, and rationale for therapy. Am J Cardiol 2003;91:2D–8D.

3. Khazanie P, Liang L, Qualls LG, et al. Outcomes of medicare beneficiaries with heart failure and atrial fibrillation. JACC Heart Fail 2014;2:41–8.

4. Dorian P, Jung W, Newman D, et al. The impairment of health-related quality of life in patients with intermittent atrial fibrillation: implications for the assessment of investigational therapy. J Am Coll Cardiol 2000;36:1303–9.

5. Chan PS, Soto G, Jones PG, et al. Patient health status and costs in heart failure: insights from the eplerenone post-acute myocardial infarction heart failure efficacy and survival study (EPHESUS). Circulation 2009;119:398–407.

6. Hoekstra T, Jaarsma T, van Veldhuisen DJ, et al. Quality of life and survival in patients with heart failure. Eur J Heart Fail 2013;15:94–102.

7. Heidenreich PA, Spertus JA, Jones PG, et al. Health status identifies heart failure outpatients at risk for hospitalization or death. J Am Coll Cardiol 2006; 47:752–6.

8. de Leon CF, Grady KL, Eaton C, et al. Quality of life in a diverse population of patients with heart failure: baseline findings from the heart failure adherence and retention trial (HART). J Cardiopulm Rehabil Prev 2009;29:171–8.

9. Olsson LG, Swedberg K, Ducharme A, et al. Atrial fibrillation and risk of clinical events in chronic heart failure with and without left ventricular systolic dysfunction: results from the Candesartan in Heart failure-Assessment of Reduction in Mortality and morbidity (CHARM) program. J Am Coll Cardiol 2006;47:1997–2004.

10. Suman-Horduna I, Roy D, Frasure-Smith N, et al. Quality of life and functional capacity in patients with atrial fibrillation and congestive heart failure. J Am Coll Cardiol 2013;61:455–60.

11. Wozakowska-Kaplon B, Opolski G. Improvement in exercise performance after successful cardioversion in patients with persistent atrial fibrillation and symptoms of heart failure. Kardiol Pol 2003;59: 213–23.

12. Guidance for industry: patient-reported outcome measures: use in medical product development to support labeling claims: draft guidance. Health Qual Life Outcomes 2006;4:79.

13. Arribas F, Ormaetxe JM, Peinado R, et al. Validation of the AF-QoL, a disease-specific quality of life questionnaire for patients with atrial fibrillation. Europace 2010;12:364–70.

14. Spertus J, Dorian P, Bubien R, et al. Development and validation of the atrial fibrillation effect on quality-of-life (AFEQT) questionnaire in patients with atrial fibrillation. Circ Arrhythm Electrophysiol 2011;4:15–25.

15. Dorian P, Guerra PG, Kerr CR, et al. Validation of a new simple scale to measure symptoms in atrial fibrillation: the Canadian Cardiovascular Society Severity in Atrial Fibrillation scale. Circ Arrhythm Electrophysiol 2009;2:218–24.

16. Wokhlu A, Monahan KH, Hodge DO, et al. Long-term quality of life after ablation of atrial fibrillation the impact of recurrence, symptom relief, and placebo effect. J Am Coll Cardiol 2010;55:2308–16.

17. Jenkins LS, Brodsky M, Schron E, et al. Quality of life in atrial fibrillation: the atrial fibrillation follow-up investigation of rhythm management (AFFIRM) study. Am Heart J 2005;149:112–20.

18. Mark DB. Assessing quality-of-life outcomes in cardiovascular clinical research. Nat Rev Cardiol 2016;13:286–308.

19. Ferreira JP, Duarte K, Graves TL, et al. Natriuretic peptides, 6-min walk test, and quality-of-life questionnaires as clinically meaningful endpoints in HF trials. J Am Coll Cardiol 2016;68:2690–707.

20. Rector TS, Francis GS, Cohn JN. Patients' self-assessment of their congestive heart failure. Part 1: patient perceived dysfunction and its poor correlation with maximal exercise tests. Heart Fail 1987;3: 192–6.

21. Rector TS, Kubo SH, Cohn JN. Patients' self-assessment of their congestive heart failure. Part 2: content, reliability and validity of a new measure, the Minnesota Living with Heart Failure Questionnaire. Heart Fail 1987;3:198–209.

22. Rector TS, Cohn JN. Assessment of patient outcome with the Minnesota Living with Heart Failure questionnaire: reliability and validity during a randomized, double-blind, placebo-controlled trial of pimobendan. Pimobendan Multicenter Research Group. Am Heart J 1992;124:1017–25.

23. Rector TS, Tschumperlin LK, Kubo SH, et al. Use of the Living with Heart Failure questionnaire to ascertain patients' perspectives on improvement in quality of life versus risk of drug-induced death. J Card Fail 1995;1:201–6.

24. Green CP, Porter CB, Bresnahan DR, et al. Development and evaluation of the Kansas City Cardiomyopathy Questionnaire: a new health status measure for heart failure. J Am Coll Cardiol 2000 35:1245–55.

25. Medical device development tool (MDDT) qualification decision summary for Kansas City cardiomyopathy questionnaire (KCCQ). Washington, DC: Food and Drug Administration; 2016.

26. Spertus JA, Jones PG. Development and validation of a short version of the Kansas City cardiomyopathy questionnaire. Circ Cardiovasc Qual Outcomes 2015;8:469–76.

27. Stehlik J, Rodriguez-Correa C, Spertus JA, et al. Implementation of real-time assessment of patient-reported outcomes in a heart failure clinic: a feasibility study. J Card Fail 2017;23:813–6.

28. Rumsfeld JS, Jones PG, Whooley MA, et al. Depression predicts mortality and hospitalization in patients with myocardial infarction complicated by heart failure. Am Heart J 2005;150:961–7.

29. Soto GE, Jones P, Weintraub WS, et al. Prognostic value of health status in patients with heart failure after acute myocardial infarction. Circulation 2004; 110:546–51.

30. Stehlik J, Estep JD, Selzman CH, et al. Patient-reported health-related quality of life is a predictor of outcomes in ambulatory heart failure patients treated with left ventricular assist device compared with medical management: results from the ROADMAP study (risk assessment and comparative effectiveness of left ventricular assist device and medical management). Circ Heart Fail 2017;10 [pii:e003910].

31. Wyse DG, Waldo AL, DiMarco JP, et al. A comparison of rate control and rhythm control in patients with atrial fibrillation. N Engl J Med 2002;347:1825–33.

32. Lumer GB, Roy D, Talajic M, et al. Amiodarone reduces procedures and costs related to atrial fibrillation in a controlled clinical trial. Eur Heart J 2002;23: 1050–6.

33. Dorian P, Mangat I. Quality of life variables in the selection of rate versus rhythm control in patients with atrial fibrillation: observations from the Canadian trial of atrial fibrillation. Card Electrophysiol Rev 2003;7:276–9.

34. Dorian P, Paquette M, Newman D, et al. Quality of life improves with treatment in the Canadian trial of atrial fibrillation. Am Heart J 2002;143:984–90.

35. Jais P, Cauchemez B, Macle L, et al. Catheter ablation versus antiarrhythmic drugs for atrial fibrillation: the A4 study. Circulation 2008;118:2498–505.

36. Wazni OM, Marrouche NF, Martin DO, et al. Radiofrequency ablation vs antiarrhythmic drugs as first-line treatment of symptomatic atrial fibrillation: a randomized trial. JAMA 2005;293:2634–40.

37. Packer DL, Mark DB, Robb RA, et al. Catheter ablation versus antiarrhythmic drug therapy for atrial fibrillation (CABANA) trial: study rationale and design. Am Heart J 2018;199:192–9.

38. Bjorkenheim A, Brandes A, Magnuson A, et al. Patient-reported outcomes in relation to continuously monitored rhythm before and during 2 years after atrial fibrillation ablation using a disease-specific and a generic instrument. J Am Heart Assoc 2018; 7 [pii:e008362].

39. Spertus J, Peterson E, Conard MW, et al. Monitoring clinical changes in patients with heart failure: a comparison of methods. Am Heart J 2005;150:707–15.

40. Ostman C, Jewiss D, Smart NA. The effect of exercise training intensity on quality of life in heart failure patients: a systematic review and meta-analysis. Cardiology 2017;136:79–89.

41. Chandra A, Lewis EF, Claggett BL, et al. Effects of sacubitril/valsartan on physical and social activity limitations in patients with heart failure: a secondary analysis of the PARADIGM-HF trial. JAMA Cardiol 2018;3:498–505.

42. Rogers JG, Aaronson KD, Boyle AJ, et al. Continuous flow left ventricular assist device improves functional capacity and quality of life of advanced heart failure patients. J Am Coll Cardiol 2010;55: 1826–34.

43. Zannad F, McMurray JJ, Krum H, et al. Eplerenone in patients with systolic heart failure and mild symptoms. N Engl J Med 2011;364:11–21.

44. McMurray JJ, Packer M, Desai AS, et al. Angiotensin-neprilysin inhibition versus enalapril in heart failure. N Engl J Med 2014;371:993–1004.

45. Trulock KM, Narayan SM, Piccini JP. Rhythm control in heart failure patients with atrial fibrillation: contemporary challenges including the role of ablation. J Am Coll Cardiol 2014;64:710–21.

46. Roy D, Talajic M, Nattel S, et al. Rhythm control versus rate control for atrial fibrillation and heart failure. N Engl J Med 2008;358:2667–77.

47. Di Biase L, Mohanty P, Mohanty S, et al. Ablation versus amiodarone for treatment of persistent atrial fibrillation in patients with congestive heart failure and an implanted device: results from the AATAC multicenter randomized trial. Circulation 2016;133:1637–44.

48. Jones DG, Haldar SK, Hussain W, et al. A randomized trial to assess catheter ablation versus rate control in the management of persistent atrial fibrillation in heart failure. J Am Coll Cardiol 2013;61:1894–903.

49. Prabhu S, Taylor AJ, Costello BT, et al. Catheter ablation versus medical rate control in atrial fibrillation and systolic dysfunction: the CAMERA-MRI study. J Am Coll Cardiol 2017;70:1949–61.

50. Marrouche NF, Brachmann J, Andresen D, et al. Catheter ablation for atrial fibrillation with heart failure. N Engl J Med 2018;378:417–27.

51. Ma Y, Bai F, Qin F, et al. Catheter ablation for treatment of patients with atrial fibrillation and heart failure: a meta-analysis of randomized controlled trials. BMC Cardiovasc Disord 2018;18:165.

52. Briceno DF, Markman TM, Lupercio F, et al. Catheter ablation versus conventional treatment of atrial fibrillation in patients with heart failure with reduced ejection fraction: a systematic review and meta-analysis of randomized controlled trials. J Interv Card Electrophysiol 2018;53:19–29.

53. Nerheim P, Birger-Botkin S, Piracha L, et al. Heart failure and sudden death in patients with tachycardia-induced cardiomyopathy and recurrent tachycardia. Circulation 2004;110:247–52.

54. Packer DL, Bardy GH, Worley SJ, et al. Tachycardia-induced cardiomyopathy: a reversible form of left ventricular dysfunction. Am J Cardiol 1986;57: 563–70.

55. Calvo N, Bisbal F, Guiu E, et al. Impact of atrial fibrillation-induced tachycardiomyopathy in patients undergoing pulmonary vein isolation. Int J Cardiol 2013;168:4093–7.

56. Bjorkenheim A, Brandes A, Magnuson A, et al. Assessment of atrial fibrillation-specific symptoms before and 2 years after atrial fibrillation ablation: do patients and physicians differ in their perception of symptom relief? JACC Clin Electrophysiol 2017;3: 1168–76.

57. Freeman JV, Simon DN, Go AS, et al. Association between atrial fibrillation symptoms, quality of life, and patient outcomes: results from the outcomes registry for better informed treatment of atrial fibrillation (ORBIT-AF). Circ Cardiovasc Qual Outcomes 2015;8:393–402.

58. Vermond RA, Crijns HJ, Tijssen JG, et al. Symptom severity is associated with cardiovascular outcome in patients with permanent atrial fibrillation in the RACE II study. Europace 2014;16:1417–25.

59. Groenveld HF, Crijns HJ, Van den Berg MP, et al. The effect of rate control on quality of life in patients with permanent atrial fibrillation: data from the RACE II (Rate Control Efficacy in Permanent Atrial Fibrillation II) study. J Am Coll Cardiol 2011;58:1795–803.

60. Mont L, Bisbal F, Hernandez-Madrid A, et al. Catheter ablation vs. antiarrhythmic drug treatment of persistent atrial fibrillation: a multicentre, randomized, controlled trial (SARA study). Eur Heart J 2014;35:501–7.

61. Bubien RS, Knotts-Dolson SM, Plumb VJ, et al. Effect of radiofrequency catheter ablation on health-related quality of life and activities of daily living in patients with recurrent arrhythmias. Circulation 1996;94:1585–91.

62. Walfridsson U, Arestedt K, Stromberg A. Development and validation of a new Arrhythmia-Specific questionnaire in Tachycardia and Arrhythmia (ASTA) with focus on symptom burden. Health Qual Life Outcomes 2012;10:44.

63. Charitakis E, Barmano N, Walfridsson U, et al. Factors predicting arrhythmia-related symptoms and health-related quality of life in patients referred for radiofrequency ablation of atrial fibrillation: an observational study (the SMURF study). JACC Clin Electrophysiol 2017;3:494–502.

64. Mark DB, Knight JD, Velazquez EJ, et al. Quality of life and economic outcomes with surgical ventricular reconstruction in ischemic heart failure: results from the surgical treatment for ischemic heart failure trial. Am Heart J 2009;157:837–44, 844.e1-3.

65. Hamo CE, Heitner JF, Pfeffer MA, et al. Baseline distribution of participants with depression and impaired quality of life in the treatment of preserved cardiac function heart failure with an aldosterone antagonist trial. Circ Heart Fail 2015;8:268–77.

66. Rector TS, Kubo SH, Cohn JN. Validity of the Minnesota Living with Heart Failure questionnaire as a measure of therapeutic response to enalapril or placebo. Am J Cardiol 1993;71:1106–7.

67. Taylor AL, Ziesche S, Yancy C, et al. Combination of isosorbide dinitrate and hydralazine in blacks with heart failure. N Engl J Med 2004;351:2049–57.

# Imaging for Risk Stratification in Atrial Fibrillation with Heart Failure

Kennosuke Yamashita, MD, PhD[a,b],
Ravi Ranjan, MD, PhD[a,b,c],*

## KEYWORDS

- Atrial fibrillation • Heart failure • Echocardiography • Computed tomography • Cardiac MRI

## KEY POINTS

- Echocardiography is a useful tool in patients with suspected heart failure, in terms of availability, safety, and cost.
- Computed tomography has the highest spatial resolution and provides detailed anatomy and functional information.
- Cardiac magnetic resonance can provide accurate anatomic and functional information and is unique in providing preoperative atrial tissue structural remodeling information and postoperative atrial scar assessment.

## INTRODUCTION
### Current Guideline

Atrial fibrillation (AF) and heart failure (HF) are associated with similar risk factors and are often present concomitantly.[1,2] AF is a potent risk factor for adverse clinical outcomes in patients with HF with preserved ejection fraction (HFpEF) or HF with reduced ejection fraction (HFrEF).[3] However, there are no specific recommendations for patients with AF with HF in the current American College of Cardiology Foundation (ACCF)/American Heart Association (AHA) and European Society Of Cardiology (ESC) guidelines (**Fig. 1**).[4,5] The main recommended goals of therapy for patients with AF with HF continue to focus on the prevention of thromboembolism and symptom relief.

Per the guidelines, rate control and rhythm control are considered at par in patients with HF who develop AF, because rhythm control therapy has not been shown to be superior to a rate control therapy.[6] As a result, catheter ablation is still considered as a second-line therapy. In contrast, for patients who develop HF following AF, per the guidelines an aggressive rhythm control strategy should be considered because in patients who have newly developed HF in the presence of AF with rapid ventricular response the likely cause is tachycardia-induced cardiomyopathy.

### Role of Imaging Modality

Cardiac imaging modalities play an important role in the diagnosis of underlying structural

Disclosure: R. Ranjan is supported by NIH grant R01HL142913 and is a consultant to Medtronic. He has or has recently had research grants from Medtronic, St Jude, and Biosense Webster. K. Yamashita has nothing to disclose.
a Division of Cardiovascular Medicine, Department of Internal Medicine, University of Utah, 30 N 1900 E, Room 4A100, Salt Lake City, Utah 84132, USA; b Nora Eccles Harrison Cardiovascular Research and Training Institute, University of Utah, 95 South 2000 East, Salt Lake City, UT 84112, USA; c Department of Biomedical Engineering, University of Utah, 36 S. Wasatch Drive, Rm. 3100, Salt Lake City, UT 84112, USA
* Corresponding author. Cardiovascular Medicine, University of Utah, 30 North 1900 East Room 4A100, Salt Lake City, UT 84132-2101.
E-mail address: ravi.ranjan@hsc.utah.edu

Cardiol Clin 37 (2019) 147–156
https://doi.org/10.1016/j.ccl.2019.01.007
0733-8651/19/© 2019 Elsevier Inc. All rights reserved.

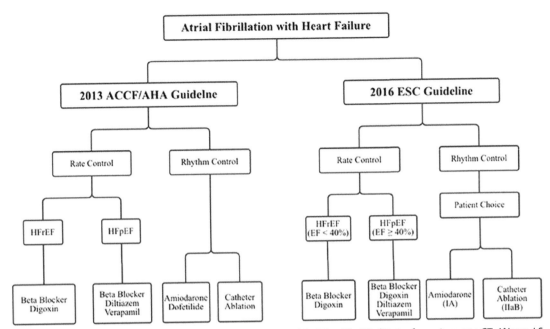

**Fig. 1.** Current guidelines for management of patients with AF with HF. (*Data from* January CT, Wann LS, Alpert JS, et al. American College of Cardiology/American Heart Association Task Force on Practice Guidelines. 2014 AHA/ACC/HRS guideline for the management of patients with atrial fibrillation: a report of the American College of Cardiology/American Heart Association Task Force on Practice Guidelines and the Heart Rhythm Society. Circulation 2014;130:e199–267; and Kirchhof P, Benussi S, Kotecha D, et al. 2016 ESC guidelines for the management of atrial fibrillation developed in collaboration with EACTS. Eur Heart J 2016;37:2893–962.)

heart disease, if any, that may cause HF and aid in guiding treatment of patients with AF. The use of a particular imaging modality should be based on the information being sought from a clinical decision-making perspective. The use of the different imaging modalities from an AF and HF perspective are briefly outlined here.

## Echocardiography

Among the different imaging modalities, echocardiography is the most commonly used and a very useful tool in patients with suspected HF, in terms of availability, safety, and cost.[7] In particular, transthoracic echocardiography (TTE) is the most common tool used in the assessment of cardiac systolic and diastolic function as well as chamber sizes of both the atria and the ventricles.[8] Transesophageal echocardiography is not routinely used to assess HF but it can be a valuable tool in patients with valvular heart disease, congenital heart disease, and suspected intracardiac thrombi in patients with AF requiring cardioversion or catheter ablation.

## Cardiac Computed Tomography

Cardiac computed tomography (CT) in patients with HF is mainly used as a noninvasive way to visualize the coronary anatomy and its severity to exclude the diagnosis of coronary artery disease. Moreover, perfusion CT may have the potential to distinguish abnormal voltage areas from normal tissue.[9] The high spatial resolution provides a detailed cardiac structure, and four-dimensional CT can provide left atrial (LA) fractional change and LA ejection fraction (EF), which are well correlated with cardiac MRI (CMR) (**Fig. 2**). It is less invasive than coronary angiography but higher level of x-ray exposure is an issue, although that seems to be getting better with improvement in technology.[10] Also, the iodinated contrast medium may induce acute kidney injury so care is needed when using this on a routine basis.[11,12]

## Cardiac MRI

CMR is well known as the gold standard for the measurements of volume, muscle mass

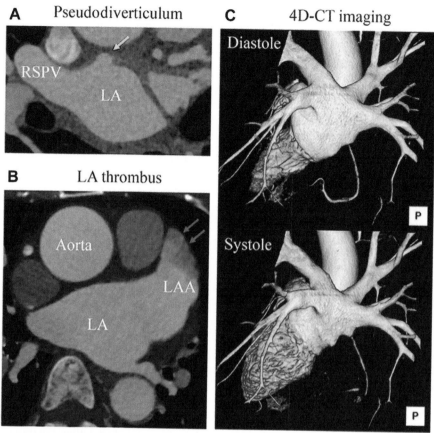

**Fig. 2.** Abnormal intracardiac structure and four-dimensional CT imaging. (*A*) Pseudodiverticulum located in LA anterior wall (*yellow arrow*). (*B*) Low-attenuation zone suspected LA thrombus (*red arrows*) is detected in left atrial appendage (LAA). (*C*) Right panel shows four-dimensional CT imaging with the ability to measure the LA function accurately. The 2 snapshots show the LA in diastole and systole. RSPV, right superior pulmonary vein.

and EF. Moreover, CMR is unique in being the imaging modality that can assess myocardial fibrosis and scar using late gadolinium enhancement (LGE). Quantitative T1 mapping has also been used to assess the extracellular volume using CMR. CMR is also useful in establishing the cause of HF and to distinguish between ischemic versus nonischemic cardiomyopathy.[13,14] In addition, CMR may be able to predict the tachycardia-induced cardiomyopathy by estimating right ventricular dysfunction.[15] The limited availability of CMR, the higher expertise required for some of these assessments, and cost are some of the limitations preventing broader use of CMR in these situations. In addition, there are other limitations, such as patients with metallic implants, claustrophobia, and severe chronic kidney disease, who are not good candidates.

## Prediction of Heart Failure in Patients with Atrial Fibrillation

Structural tissue remodeling, including increased collagen disposition, loss of myocytes, and fibrosis, has been shown to be related to AF.[16] Azadani and colleagues[17] reported the higher levels of LA fibrosis detected by LGE-CMR in patients who subsequently developed HF. Left ventricular fibrosis measured by two-dimensional echocardiography using integrated backscatter might contribute to left ventricular diastolic dysfunction and the high prevalence of HFpEF in patients with AF.[18] Moreover, not only older age but also LA pressure greater than or equal to 11 mm Hg, and peak systolic mitral annular velocity less than or equal to 9.3 cm/s measured by TTE were independent predictors of early HFpEF.[19] In patients who developed new-onset HF, 80% were found to have a preserved left ventricular EF and were classified as having HFpEF. More studies are needed to confirm the definition of early HF using imaging.

### Prediction of Atrial Fibrillation in Patients with Heart Failure

Several studies have reported the prediction of AF in patients with HF using different imaging modalities and measurement. The substudy from the TOPCAT study showed that decreased peak A-wave velocity measured by TTE was positively correlated with the risk of AF in patients with HFpEF.[20] The diastolic parameter of LA function was possibly a more important tool in AF risk assessment than LA dilatation, such as large LA area and volume. Also, left ventricular filling pressure measured by TTE was reported as a good predictor of new-onset AF in patients with HF.[21] Noninvasive evaluation of the total atrial conduction time measured by tissue Doppler imaging has also been reported to be a useful tool in predicting AF occurrence in patients with HF.[22] Moreover, in terms of AF occurrence in patients with HFrEF, several studies have reported that echocardiography parameters such as LA size are a well-accepted risk factor for AF.[23,24]

### Predicting Future Cardiac Events in Patients with Heart Failure with Atrial Fibrillation

AF is a potential risk factor for adverse clinical outcomes with HFpEF or HFrEF.[3] Regardless of the EF, the presence and extent of LGE enhancement identified by CMR is an independent predictor of major adverse cardiac events in patients with AF.[25] Even in cardiac resynchronization therapy (CRT) recipients, patients who develop new-onset AF had less echocardiographic response to CRT and more adverse cardiac events.[26] Therefore, clinicians should focus on treatment of AF in patients with HFpEF or HFrEF and consider maintaining sinus rhythm.

### Ablation for Atrial Fibrillation with Heart Failure

Several prospective randomized control trials have shown the effectiveness of catheter ablation in patients with AF with HFrEF (**Table 1**).[27–33] In contrast, few reports are available on the impact of catheter ablation in patients with AF with HFpEF. Meta-analysis has shown significant improvement of left ventricular EF, especially, in patients with significantly reduced EF at baseline.[34,35] Recently, technological advancement

has made catheter ablation safer and more effective than before. Despite this progress, arrhythmia recurrence following catheter ablation continues to be a clinical reality and more needs to be done to improve outcomes.[36] In summary, indications for catheter ablation in patients with HFrEF with concomitant AF should be carefully evaluated preoperatively using an imaging modality and the procedures should be performed in experienced centers with experienced operators.

### Imaging Before Procedure

Atrial fibrotic change is well known to be associated with AF.[37,38] CMR has been shown to detect this preablation LA fibrosis. The atrial tissue fibrosis amount detected by LGE-CMR was independently related to arrhythmia recurrence after ablation.[39] In the subgroup of patients with extensive atrial fibrosis, arrhythmia-free survival at day 375 was only 31.6%. This result can be useful in preoperatively identifying the patients who are poor candidates for aggressive rhythm control therapy and catheter ablation. These patients with extensive LA fibrosis based on CMR also had enlarged LA, so the chamber size can also be used as a surrogate. Meanwhile, there are limitations to using CMR for LA fibrosis detection, including setting the threshold.[40] As a result, the use of CMR to detect LA fibrosis and predict ablation outcomes has not been universally reported. Sramko and colleagues[41] reported that the extent of LA-LGE did not predict AF recurrence after ablation. More recently, contrast-enhanced perfusion CT has also been reported to identify areas with low LA voltage.[9] Further studies are needed to confirm the methodology and reproduce the outcomes.

Preimaging with MRI can also be used to define both the atrial structure and structures including and surrounding the esophagus (**Fig. 3**).[42] The esophagus is a mobile structure so the preimaging location might not be useful when ablating. A recent report has shown that if the gap between the posterior wall of the LA and the vertebral body is less than 4.5 mm then the odds ratio of the esophagus not moving is 9.25 (95% confidence interval, 1.72–49.67).[4] This finding can be useful when planning for ablation to minimize any esophageal injury. **Fig. 2** also shows how the higher image resolution in CT can be used to detect small structural perturbations in the LA, which can be useful when targeting gaps to get complete pulmonary vein (PV) isolation.

**Table 1**
Randomized controlled trials for catheter ablation of atrial fibrillation in patients with heart failure with reduced ejection fraction

| Study | Multi-center | Publication Year | Sample Size | Age (y) | EF (%) | Persistent AF (%) | Mean Number of Procedures | Catheter Ablation Group | Comparison Group | Follow-up (mo) | Primary End Point | Sinus Restoration | Results |
|---|---|---|---|---|---|---|---|---|---|---|---|---|---|
| PABA-CHF[27] | Yes | 2008 | 81 | 60 | 27 | 51.0 | 1.2 | PVI (41) | AV node ablation with biventricular pacing (40) | 6 | Composite of post, 6-MWD and MLWHF score | 71% without AAD | Catheter ablation was superior to AV nodal ablation and biventricular pacing |
| MacDonald et al,[28] | No | 2011 | 41 | 64 | 15.1 | 100 | 1.35 | PVI ± linear ± CFAE (22) | Rate control (19) | 6 | LVEF measured by CMR | 50% | No significant difference between groups |
| ARC-HF[29] | No | 2013 | 52 | 64 | 22 | 100 | 1.23 | PVI ± linear ± CFAE (26) | Rate control (26) | 12 | Peak $Vo_2$ | 88% without AAD | Improvement in peak $Vo_2$ in the catheter ablation group compared with rate control |
| CAMTAF[30] | No | 2014 | 50 | 55 | 31.8 | 100 | 1.7 | PVI ± linear ± CFAE (26) | Rate control (24) | 12 | LVEF at 6 mo | 81% at 6 mo 73% at 1 y | Improvement in LVEF at 6 mo in catheter ablation group |

(continued on next page)

**Table 1** (*continued*)

| Study | Multi-center | Publication Year | Sample Size | Age (y) | EF (%) | Persistent AF (%) | Mean Number of Procedures | Catheter Ablation Group | Comparison Group | Follow-up (mo) | Primary End Point | Sinus Restoration | Results |
|---|---|---|---|---|---|---|---|---|---|---|---|---|---|
| AATAC[31] | Yes | 2016 | 203 | 62 | 29 | 100 | 1.4 | PVI ± posterior wall ± CFAE (102) | Amiodarone (101) | 36 | Freedom from AF | 70% | Significant improvement in freedom from AF in the catheter ablation group |
| CAMERA-CMR[32] | Yes | 2017 | 68 | 59 | 34 | 100 | NA | PVI + posterior wall (34) | Rate control (34) | 6 | LVEF measured by CMR | 100% using DCCV | Significant improvement in EF in catheter ablation group |
| CASTLE-AF[33] | Yes | 2018 | 363 | 64 | 32.5 | 70.0 | 1.3 | PVI ± linear ± CFAE (179) | Medical rate or rhythm control (184) | 60 | Death or HF hospitalization | 63% | Significant improvement in composite end point of death and HF hospitalization in catheter ablation group |

*Abbreviations:* AV, atrioventricular; AAD, antiarrhythmic drugs; CFAE, complex fractionated atrial electrograms; DCCV, direct-current cardioversion; LVEF, left ventricular EF; MLWHF, Minnesota living with heart failure; PVI, pulmonary vein isolation; 6-MWD, 6-minute walk distance; $Vo_2$, oxygen uptake.

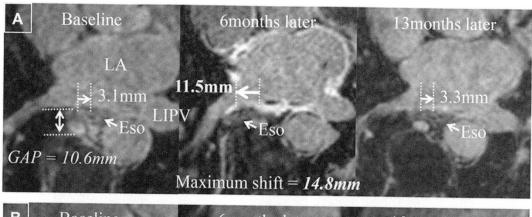

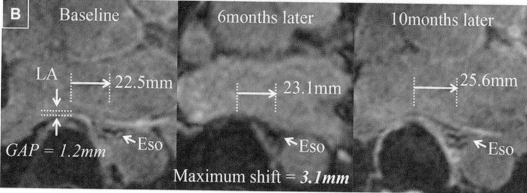

**Fig. 3.** Use of MRI to predict esophageal position during ablation. (*A*) Patient with a gap of 10.6 mm having 14.8 mm of esophageal movement. (*B*) Patient with a gap of 1.2 mm having only 3.1 mm of esophageal movement. Eso, esophagus; LIPV, left inferior pulmonary vein.

## Imaging During Procedures

Intracardiac echocardiography (ICE) is used to provide high-resolution real-time visualization of cardiac structures and catheter location, and early recognition of procedural complications. Recently, a three-dimensional (3D) ICE system has also been developed and has the advantage of providing additional anatomic detail. In particular, 3D ICE systems can monitor the esophageal position and the proximity to the esophagus.[43] In contrast, real-time CMR has the potential to detect an occluded PV with balloon, lesion formation, and potentially even collateral damage.[44,45] Moreover, real-time CMR may be able to detect gaps in a liner lesion set, allowing them to be targeted right away.[46] However, CMR-compatible devices need to be implemented before this becomes a clinical reality.

## Imaging After Procedure

LGE-CMR has been used to estimate chronic lesion scarring after radiofrequency ablation in the LA (**Fig. 4**).[46] Real-time monitoring of tip-to-tissue contact force has improved clinical outcomes and decreased complications, but insufficient tissue injury and ablation-related edema formation are thought to be the main causes of reversible electrical conduction and arrhythmia recurrence.[47,48] Acute edema related to radiofrequency ablation resolves over the span of few weeks and higher contact force has been shown to be related to creation of larger edema,[49,50] but a different power source could make a chronic scar with less acute edema.[51] Catheter ablation of AF targeting the PVs rarely achieves permanent encircling of the PV with scar, and this has been shown to affect clinical outcomes.[47,52] Hence, more experimental and clinical studies are needed to develop the best means of lesion creation while minimizing the creation of reversible edema. Postablation LGE-MRI can be used to visualize ablation-induced scarring and identify gaps in lesion sets (see **Fig. 4**), which can be useful when planning redo ablations.

## Axial view of LGE-CMR

## 3D scar imaging

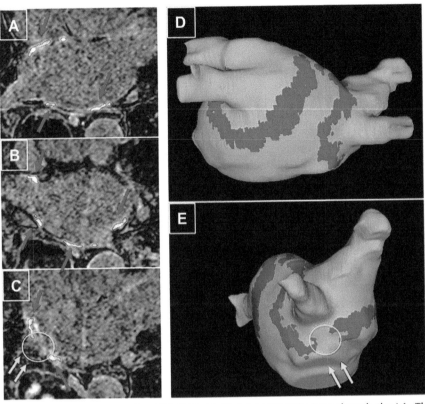

**Fig. 4.** Postablation LA scar imaging using LGE-CMR. (*A–C*) Axial LGE-MRI views though the LA. The scar areas have higher image intensity. 3D PA view (*D*) and right lateral (*E*) view of the LA showing scar along the PVs. In LGE-CMR axial views, the areas of enhancement are segmented (*red arrows*) and are shown as scar (*red areas*) in the 3D image. The gap between scar areas can be seen both in axial and 3D right lateral images (gap is marked with the yellow arrows).

## SUMMARY

Cardiac imaging plays an important role in the assessment of anatomic structure and cardiac function. New imaging technology and techniques have been developed that provide more precise assessment of the underlying myocardial substrate and can be useful in predicting the risk of AF in patients with HF. Moreover, imaging modalities are able to identify preablation atrial fibrosis and scar formation following catheter ablation. Studies are needed to further validate the new techniques and define the usefulness of these additional imaging techniques, but they hold immense promise in AF risk prediction, improving patient selection for ablation, and improving ablation outcomes.

## REFERENCES

1. Balasubramaniam R, Kistler PM. Atrial fibrillation in heart failure: the chicken or the egg? Heart 2009; 95:535–9.

2. Kotecha D, Piccini JP. Atrial fibrillation in heart failure what should we do? Eur Heart J 2015;36:3250–7.

3. Lubitz SA, Lunetta KL, Lin H, et al. Novel genetic markers associate with atrial fibrillation risk in Europeans and Japanese. J Am Coll Cardiol 2014;63: 1200–10.

4. January CT, Wann LS, Alpert JS, et al. 2014 AHA/ACC/HRS guideline for the management of patients with atrial fibrillation: a report of the American College of Cardiology/American Heart Association Task Force on Practice Guidelines and the Heart Rhythm Society. Circulation 2014;130:e199–267.

5. Kirchhof P, Benussi S, Kotecha D, et al. 2016 ESC guidelines for the management of atrial fibrillation developed in collaboration with EACTS. Eur Heart J 2016;37:2893–962.

6. Roy D, Talajic M, Nattel S, et al. Rhythm control versus rate control for atrial fibrillation and heart failure. N Engl J Med 2008;358:2667–77.

7. Parvez B, Vaglio J, Rowan S, et al. Symptomatic response to antiarrhythmic drug therapy

modulated by a common single nucleotide polymorphism in atrial fibrillation. J Am Coll Cardiol 2012;60: 539–45.

8. Benjamin Shoemaker M, Muhammad R, Parvez B, et al. Common atrial fibrillation risk alleles at 4q25 predict recurrence after catheter-based atrial fibrillation ablation. Heart Rhythm 2013;10: 394–400.

9. Ling Z, McManigle J, Zipunnikov V, et al. The association of left atrial low-voltage regions on electroanatomic mapping with low attenuation regions on cardiac computed tomography perfusion imaging in patients with atrial fibrillation. Heart Rhythm 2015;12:857–64.

10. Kuhl JT, Lonborg J, Fuchs A, et al. Assessment of left atrial volume and function: a comparative study between echocardiography, magnetic resonance imaging and multi slice computed tomography. Int J Cardiovasc Imaging 2012;28:1061–71.

11. Rear R, Bell RM, Hausenloy DJ. Contrast-induced nephropathy following angiography and cardiac interventions. Heart 2016;102:638–48.

12. Yamashita K, Igawa W, Ono M, et al. Safety and efficacy of tolvaptan for prevention of contrast-induced acute kidney injury in patients with heart failure and chronic kidney disease. Kidney Dis 2018. https://doi.org/10.1159/000494724.

13. Gramley F, Lorenzen J, Plisiene J, et al. Decreased plasminogen activator inhibitor and tissue metalloproteinase inhibitor expression may promote increased metalloproteinase activity with increasing duration of human atrial fibrillation. J Cardiovasc Electrophysiol 2007;18:1076–82.

14. Barretto AC, Mady C, Nussbacher A, et al. Atrial fibrillation in endomyocardial fibrosis is a marker of worse prognosis. Int J Cardiol 1998;67:19–25.

15. Okada A, Nakajima I, Morita Y, et al. Diagnostic value of right ventricular dysfunction in tachycardia-induced cardiomyopathy using cardiac magnetic resonance imaging. Circ J 2016;80:2141–8.

16. Ausma J, Wijffels M, Thone F, et al. Structural changes of atrial myocardium due to sustained atrial fibrillation in the goat. Circulation 1997;96: 3157–63.

17. Azadani PN, King JB, Kheirkhahan M, et al. Left atrial fibrosis is associated with new-onset heart failure in patients with atrial fibrillation. Int J Cardiol 2017;248:161–5.

18. Shantsila E, Shantsila A, Blann AD, et al. Left ventricular fibrosis in atrial fibrillation. Am J Cardiol 2013; 111:996–1001.

19. Meluzin J, Starek Z, Kulik T, et al. Prevalence and predictors of early heart failure with preserved ejection fraction in patients with paroxysmal atrial fibrillation. J Card Fail 2017;23:558–62.

20. O'Neal WT, Sandesara P, Patel N, et al. Echocardiographic predictors of atrial fibrillation in patients with heart failure with preserved ejection fraction. Eur Heart J Cardiovasc Imaging 2017;18:725–9.

21. Mornos C, Petrescu L, Cozma D, et al. A new tissue Doppler index in predicting future atrial fibrillation in patients with heart failure. Arq Bras Cardiol 2011;97: 468–77.

22. Bertini M, Borleffs CJ, Delgado V, et al. Prediction of atrial fibrillation in patients with an implantable cardioverter-defibrillator and heart failure. Eur J Heart Fail 2010;12:1101–10.

23. Bonapace S, Rossi A, Cicoira M, et al. Echocardiographically derived pulse wave velocity and diastolic dysfunction are associated with an increased incidence of atrial fibrillation in patients with systolic heart failure. Echocardiography 2016;33:1024–31.

24. Kato TS, Di Tullio MR, Qian M, et al. Clinical and echocardiographic factors associated with new-onset atrial fibrillation in heart failure –subanalysis of the WARCEF trial. Circ J 2016;80:619–26.

25. Suksaranjit P, McGann CJ, Akoum N, et al. Prognostic implications of left ventricular scar determined by late gadolinium enhanced cardiac magnetic resonance in patients with atrial fibrillation. Am J Cardiol 2016;118:991–7.

26. Borleffs CJ, Ypenburg C, van Bommel RJ, et al. Clinical importance of new-onset atrial fibrillation after cardiac resynchronization therapy. Heart Rhythm 2009;6:305–10.

27. Khan MN, Jais P, Cummings J, et al. Pulmonary-vein isolation for atrial fibrillation in patients with heart failure. N Engl J Med 2008;359:1778–85.

28. MacDonald MR, Connelly DT, Hawkins NM, et al. Radiofrequency ablation for persistent atrial fibrillation in patients with advanced heart failure and severe left ventricular systolic dysfunction: a randomised controlled trial. Heart 2011;97: 740–7.

29. Jones DG, Haldar SK, Hussain W, et al. A randomized trial to assess catheter ablation versus rate control in the management of persistent atrial fibrillation in heart failure. J Am Coll Cardiol 2013;61:1894–903.

30. Hunter RJ, Berriman TJ, Diab I, et al. A randomized controlled trial of catheter ablation versus medical treatment of atrial fibrillation in heart failure (the CAMTAF trial). Circ Arrhythm Electrophysiol 2014; 7:31–8.

31. Di Biase L, Mohanty P, Mohanty S, et al. Ablation versus amiodarone for treatment of persistent atrial fibrillation in patients with congestive heart failure and an implanted device: results from the AATAC multicenter randomized trial. Circulation 2016;133: 1637–44.

32. Prabhu S, Taylor AJ, Costello BT, et al. Catheter ablation versus medical rate control in atrial fibrillation and systolic dysfunction: the

CAMERA-MRI study. J Am Coll Cardiol 2017;70:
1949–61.

33. Marrouche NF, Brachmann J, Andresen D, et al.
Catheter ablation for atrial fibrillation with heart failure. N Engl J Med 2018;378:417–27.

34. Anselmino M, Matta M, D'Ascenzo F, et al. Catheter
ablation of atrial fibrillation in patients with left ventricular systolic dysfunction: a systematic review
and meta-analysis. Circ Arrhythm Electrophysiol
2014;7:1011–8.

35. Zhu M, Zhou X, Cai H, et al. Catheter ablation
versus medical rate control for persistent atrial
fibrillation in patients with heart failure: a
PRISMA-compliant systematic review and meta-
analysis of randomized controlled trials. Medicine
2016;95:e4377.

36. Ouyang F, Antz M, Ernst S, et al. Recovered pulmonary vein conduction as a dominant factor for
recurrent atrial tachyarrhythmias after complete
circular isolation of the pulmonary veins: lessons
from double Lasso technique. Circulation 2005;
111:127–35.

37. Li D, Fareh S, Leung TK, et al. Promotion of atrial
fibrillation by heart failure in dogs: atrial remodeling
of a different sort. Circulation 1999;100:87–95.

38. Everett TH, Olgin JE. Atrial fibrosis and the mechanisms of atrial fibrillation. Heart Rhythm 2007;4:
S24–7.

39. Marrouche NF, Wilber D, Hindricks G, et al. Association of atrial tissue fibrosis identified by delayed
enhancement MRI and atrial fibrillation catheter
ablation: the DECAAF study. JAMA 2014;311:
498–506.

40. Appelbaum E, Manning WJ. Left atrial fibrosis by
late gadolinium enhancement cardiovascular magnetic resonance predicts recurrence of atrial fibrillation after pulmonary vein isolation: do you see what I
see? Circ Arrhythm Electrophysiol 2014;7:2–4.

41. Sramko M, Peichl P, Wichterle D, et al. Clinical value
of assessment of left atrial late gadolinium enhancement in patients undergoing ablation of atrial fibrillation. Int J Cardiol 2015;179:351–7.

42. Yamashita K, Quang C, Schroeder JD, et al. Distance between the left atrium and the vertebral
body is predictive of esophageal movement in serial
MR imaging. J Interv Card Electrophysiol 2018;52:
149–56.

43. Ren J, Callans DJ, Marchlinski FE, et al. 3D intracardiac echocardiography/cartosound imaging of
esophagus guided left atrial posterior wall ablation
for atrial fibrillation. J Atrial Fibrillation 2014;7:1184.

44. Lichter J, Kholmovski EG, Coulombe N, et al. Real-
time magnetic resonance imaging-guided cryoablation of the pulmonary veins with acute freeze-zone
and chronic lesion assessment. Europace 2019;
21(1):154–62.

45. Kholmovski EG, Coulombe N, Silvernagel J, et al.
Real-time MRI-guided cardiac cryo-ablation: a feasibility study. J Cardiovasc Electrophysiol 2016;27:
602–8.

46. Ranjan R, Kholmovski EG, Blauer J, et al. Identification and acute targeting of gaps in atrial ablation
lesion sets using a real-time magnetic resonance imaging system. Circ Arrhythm Electrophysiol 2012;5:
1130–5.

47. Parmar BR, Jarrett TR, Burgon NS, et al. Comparison of left atrial area marked ablated in electroana-
tomical maps with scar in MRI. J Cardiovasc
Electrophysiol 2014;25:457–63.

48. Ranjan R, Kato R, Zviman MM, et al. Gaps in the
ablation line as a potential cause of recovery
from electrical isolation and their visualization using MRI. Circ Arrhythm Electrophysiol 2011;4:
279–86.

49. Ghafoori E, Kholmovski EG, Thomas S, et al. Characterization of gadolinium contrast enhancement of
radiofrequency ablation lesions in predicting edema
and chronic lesion size. Circ Arrhythm Electrophysiol
2017;10 [pii:e005599].

50. Thomas S, Silvernagel J, Angel N, et al. Higher contact force during radiofrequency ablation leads to a
much larger increase in edema as compared to
chronic lesion size. J Cardiovasc Electrophysiol
2018;29:1143–9.

51. Yamashita K, Kholmovski E, Ghafoori E, et al. Characterization of edema after cryo and radiofrequency
ablation based on serial MR imaging. J Cardiovasc
Electrophysiol 2018. https://doi.org/10.1111/jce.
13785.

52. Parmar BR, Jarrett TR, Kholmovski EG, et al. Poor
scar formation after ablation is associated with atria
fibrillation recurrence. J Interv Card Electrophysio
2015;44:247–56.

# Does Left Ventricular Systolic Function Matter? Treating Atrial Fibrillation in HFrEF Versus HFpEF

Michael B. Stokes, MBBS[a],
Prashanthan Sanders, MBBS, PhD[b],*

## KEYWORDS

- Atrial fibrillation • HF-pEF • HF-rEF • Systolic function • Catheter ablation

## KEY POINTS

- Atrial fibrillation (AF) and heart failure (HF) frequently coexist and are associated with adverse outcomes compared with incidence of both respective conditions occurring individually.
- A comprehensive assessment of LV systolic function is essential in the investigation of the newly diagnosed AF patient.
- Restoration of sinus rhythm in HF patients with AF (via pharmacologic, electrical, and catheter therapies), should be pursued to avoid worsening symptoms and progression of HF in appropriately selected patients with both HF with preserved ejection fraction (HF-pEF) and HF with reduced ejection fraction (HF-rEF).
- Catheter ablation has an increasing role in AF with HF-rEF, but requires further studies in AF with HF-pEF.
- HFpEF has several variable clinical phenotypes that may have differing clinical expressions of AF and an associated spectrum of clinical progression.

## INTRODUCTION

Atrial fibrillation (AF) and heart failure (HF) are both monumental health care challenges that contribute significantly to hospitalizations, health care costs, and mortality. These 2 diseases frequently coexist and both possess numerous similar clustering risk factors. The development of AF in HF patients commonly heralds HF progression and is associated with adverse outcomes including increasing rates of HF hospitalizations, mortality, and thromboembolic events.[1,2]

Comprehensive AF management requires multiple management interventions including lifestyle,

Disclosure Statement: Dr M.B. Stokes has no disclosures for this publication. Dr P. Sanders reports having served on the advisory board of Biosense-Webster, Boston Scientific, CathRx, Medtronic, and St Jude Medical. Dr P. Sanders reports that the University of Adelaide has received on his behalf lecture and/or consulting fees from Biosense Webster (United States), Medtronic (United States), Boston-Scientific, Pfizer (United States), and St Jude Medical (United States). Dr P. Sanders reports that the University of Adelaide has received on his behalf research funding from Medtronic, St Jude Medical, Boston Scientific, Biotronik (Germany), and Liva-Nova (France).

[a] Department of Cardiology, South Australian Health and Medical Research Institute, University of Adelaide, Royal Adelaide Hospital, Port Road, Adelaide, South Australia 5000, Australia; [b] Department of Cardiology, Centre for Heart Rhythm Disorders, South Australian Health and Medical Research Institute, University of Adelaide, Royal Adelaide Hospital, Port Road, Adelaide, South Australia 5000, Australia
* Corresponding author.
*E-mail address:* prash.sanders@adelaide.edu.au

Cardiol Clin 37 (2019) 157–166
https://doi.org/10.1016/j.ccl.2019.01.008

pharmacologic, and appropriately selected electro-physiologic therapies. Among these interventions, essential management decisions in AF include the long-term rhythm strategy (either rhythm or rate control), commencement of therapeutic anticoagulation to prevent thromboembolic events, and candidacy for catheter ablation.

Regardless of the varied clinical presentations of AF, cardiac structural and functional assessment provides vital information to enable informed clinical decision making. In the initial assessment, quantification of left ventricular (LV) systolic function contributes to the clinical context. The information obtained assists in diagnosing HF with preserved ejection fraction (HF-pEF) and HF with reduced ejection fraction (HF-rEF).

This review discusses aspects of AF occurrence and management, specifically relating to HF-rEF versus HF-pEF.

## SCOPE OF THE PROBLEM

The relationship of AF and HF is complex with contributory mechanisms of both conditions to each other. HF occurring with concomitant AF is very common. In a large Swedish registry (Swede-HF) of more than 41,000 patients, the prevalence of AF in HF-rEF, HF with mid-range ejection fraction (HF-mEF), and HF-pEF was 53%, 60%, and 65% respectively. In all these HF groups, factors associated with the presence of AF included male sex, increased age, prior myocardial infarction, and prior stroke or transient ischemic attack.[1] Similarly, a large United States registry of AF patients found that development of HF was associated with significantly elevated mortality and that the rate of HF development was 20% at 5 years following the initial AF diagnosis.[3] HF-pEF is a burgeoning disease and concomitant AF developing at any point in its natural history is common, with 66% incidence of AF with HF-pEF in a large United States registry that followed HF-pEF patients for a median of 3.7 years. AF with HF-pEF was associated with significantly worse outcomes than HF-pEF with sinus rhythm.[4]

## MEASUREMENT OF LEFT VENTRICULAR SYSTOLIC FUNCTION

Comprehensive systolic function assessment via transthoracic echocardiography includes multiple parameters that measure myocardial function. These include accurate measurement of ejection fraction (via several methods), myocardial shortening (via global longitudinal strain), stroke volume assessment, and quantification of mitral annular systolic motion.[5]

Specific to AF, beat-to-beat variation and poor ventricular rate control can affect reproducibility of these parameters of systolic function. As a result, quantification of systolic function is commonly more challenging compared with patients in sinus rhythm. Additional patient factors at the time of study acquisition, including rate control and afterload, may also affect the assessment of systolic function (**Table 1**).

## SYSTOLIC FUNCTION IN HF-rEF

HF-rEF is defined by occurrence of the clinical presentation of HF, accompanied by objective evidence of reduced ejection fraction. Current international guidelines define this by a left ventricular ejection fraction (LVEF) less than 40%.[6] Of note, a new designation of HF has been recently been defined. HF-mEF is defined by LVEF of 40% to 49% and although HF-mEF has many clinical properties similar to those of HF-rEF, at this stage it is largely an attempt to stimulate research in this population of HF patients who commonly have mixed systolic and diastolic dysfunction.

## SYSTOLIC FUNCTION IN HF-pEF

Although HF-pEF is defined by the clinical presentation of HF with preserved ejection fraction (LVEF >50%),[6] several parameters of systolic function may be abnormal. Many parameters of LV diastolic function reflect a continuum with numerous systolic function variables including mitral annular systolic ejection velocity, mitral annular plane systolic descent, and LV global longitudinal strain.[5] These parameters are commonly impaired in patients with HF-pEF.

HF-pEF is a clinical syndrome with multiple and increasingly defined phenotypes. Although the simplest measure of systolic function (LVEF) may be normal in most of these patients, other abnormalities of systolic function and diastolic function are commonly identified on echocardiography. A classification of HF-pEF is presented in **Box 1**.

## DIAGNOSIS OF HF-pEF IN ATRIAL FIBRILLATION PATIENTS

As mentioned previously, the assessment of systolic function as well as intracardiac filling pressures in HF-pEF with AF is challenging, with variable cycle lengths (with beat-to-beat stroke volume variation). In addition, many HF-pEF patients demonstrate normal intracardiac filling pressures at rest, which do become elevated with exercise. Performance in a "diastolic stress test" may identify HF-pEF patients via the assessment of mitral E wave, measurement of mitral annular

**Table 1**
**Assessment of LV systolic function**

| | |
|---|---|
| Ejection fraction (TTE) | Echocardiography-derived ejection fraction (via Simpson biplane method; 3D volumes; area-length method) |
| Ejection fraction (CMR) | Cardiac MRI (accurate end-diastolic, end-systolic volume measurement) |
| LV stroke volume (TTE) | Using pulsed-wave Doppler signal and the cross-sectional area of the LV outflow tract |
| dP/dT (TTE) | Quantification of ventricular contractility, derived from continuous-wave Doppler signal of mitral regurgitation jet. Is independent of ventricular load |
| Tei index (TTE) | Marker of myocardial performance. Calculated using measurements from pulsed-wave Doppler signals positioned at the mitral inflow and LV outflow tract |
| Global longitudinal strain (TTE) | Speckle tracking of myocardial shortening across 18 myocardial segments. Provides assessment of myocardial systolic function, independent of ejection fraction. May be reduced in early systolic dysfunction and/or HF-pEF |
| Tissue Doppler imaging (TTE) | The velocity of the mitral annular plane, toward and away from the LV apex in systole and diastole, provides quantitative assessment of LV longitudinal function. S′ = systolic myocardial velocity (lateral mitral annulus); e′ = early diastolic myocardial velocity; a′ = late diastolic myocardial velocity resulting from atrial contraction (lateral mitral annulus). S′ and e′ are commonly reduced in HF-pEF without necessarily a fall in ejection fraction |

*Abbreviations*: CMR, cardiac MRI; TTE, echocardiography.

E′ velocity, and the peak tricuspid regurgitant signal following peak stress.

An increasing body of evidence suggests that HF-pEF is found in patients with paroxysmal AF more often than is commonly appreciated. This evidence is supported by a study published by Meluzin and colleagues[7] in 2017 of 115 consecutive AF patients presenting for catheter ablation. Left atrial pressure (LAP) was measured invasively following the transseptal puncture, both at rest and following arm exercise. Early HF-pEF was defined as normal LAP, but elevated LAP greater than 25 mm Hg with exercise; and advanced HF-pEF was defined as elevated resting LAP greater than 15 mm Hg. In this population of unselected, consecutive paroxysmal AF patients, 14% had HF-pEF at rest and 25% had early HF-pEF that was unmasked with exercise.

A further hemodynamic study by Reddy and colleagues[8] documented rates of HF-pEF (defined as exercise pulmonary capillary wedge pressure >25 mm Hg) in patients with "unexplained dyspnea." Consecutive right heart catheterizations with exercise were performed in a population of 429 such patients (101 of who had a history of AF). Exercise-induced HF-pEF was highly prevalent in AF patients with 98% incidence in those with a history of persistent or permanent

AF and 91% incidence in those with paroxysmal AF. Incidentally, 55% of patients with exertional dyspnea who were in sinus rhythm had evidence of exercise-induced HF-pEF.

## THE "CHICKEN AND EGG"

The conundrum of whether AF is the causation of an individual patient's HF or reflects a pathophysiologic consequence of HF is commonly contentious. AF may contribute to HF development via various pathophysiologic pathways, with 2 commonly postulated.

First, development of AF results in a loss of atrial systole (or atrial "kick"), which may impair cardiac output by up to 25%.[9] In addition, AF is associated with a reduction in other atrial functions including conduit and reservoir function (both of which facilitate drainage of pulmonary venous blood and passively fill the left ventricle), further compromising cardiac output.[10] In patients with hypertrophied fibrotic ventricles who are particularly sensitive to changes in atrial function, AF development may precipitate the clinical presentation of HF.

Second, AF may also contribute to HF via development of a "tachycardia-mediated cardiomyopathy," which can develop in persisting uncontrolled ventricular rate from AF. Persistent tachycardia

---

**Box 1**
**Phenotypic classification of HF-pEF**

1. Chronic systemic hypertension–associated HF-pEF

   Systemic hypertension, systemic factors, and vascular dysfunction → LV concentric hypertrophy and diastolic dysfunction → LV fibrosis and elevated LV filling pressure → left atrial hypertension and left atrial dysfunction

   ↓

   Pulmonary hypertension → right ventricular impairment

   ↓

   Clinical presentation of HF-pEF

2. Non–hypertension-associated HF-pEF

   - Valvular aortic and/or mitral valve disease
   - Cardiomyopathic:
     o Restrictive cardiomyopathies
     o Hypertrophic cardiomyopathies
     o Infiltrative cardiomyopathies (eg, amyloidosis, Fabry disease)
   - Extramyocardial
     o Pericardial disease
     o Left atrial dysfunction, left atrial fibrosis, "stiff left atrial syndrome"
     o Obesity phenotype

---

results in dilation of cardiac chambers, typically accompanied by thinning or preservation of wall thickness without hypertrophy. This occurs from disruption of the extracellular matrix, which can compromise myocyte alignment, with resultant chamber dilatation. Changes in myocyte structure, size, and protein synthesis have also been reported. Chronic low-grade myocardial ischemia is also a postulated mechanism in the setting of supraphysiologic heart rates and high ventricular filling pressures.[11]

In addition, several other pathophysiologic pathways may contribute to HF development with AF, including adverse neurohormonal pathway activation (via excessive angiotensin II and noradrenaline release in AF patients). Diffuse ventricular fibrosis has also been documented in chronic AF patients via postcontrast T1 mapping on cardiac magnetic resonance imaging (MRI).[12,13]

Alternatively, HF occurring primarily and AF developing consequently is also an important clinical course that develops in numerous patients. Animal HF models have reported development of atrial fibrosis and altered atrial electrical conduction (with attenuation of action potential duration) following rapid-ventricular pacing-induced HF.[14,15]

In patients with LV dysfunction (either systolic or diastolic), the consequence of chronically elevated ventricular volume and pressure overload is left atrial enlargement. In HF-pEF, hypertrophied fibrotic ventricles are poorly compliant, with transmission of the pressure to the left atrium and subsequent chamber enlargement. This also occurs in HF-rEF via both transmission of pressure and other factors that may develop, including functional mitral regurgitation because of mitral annular dilatation. Development of AF has been shown to have a linear relationship with increasing left atrial volumes, representing a clear pathway for development in the chronic HF-pEF or HF-rEF patient.[16]

In addition to the aforementioned, many of the risks for development of AF (such as obesity, hypertension, and heavy alcohol consumption) are in their own right independent risk factors for HF development.[17]

## EFFECT OF ATRIAL FIBRILLATION ON PROGNOSIS OF HF-pEF

A large HF-pEF randomized controlled study of spironolactone (the TOPCAT study) highlighted the adverse consequences of AF in a recently published subanalysis, which assessed whether AF modified the treatment response to spironolactone and whether spironolactone influenced postrandomization AF. The primary outcome of the TOPCAT study was a composite of cardiovascular mortality, aborted cardiac arrest, and hospitalization for HF. At baseline, AF was common in this study (43% overall), with 18% having a history of AF and 25% having AF on their ECG at enrollment. The presence of AF did not modify any treatment effect of spironolactone; however, AF on ECG at enrollment did increase cardiovascular risk (hazard ratio [HR] 1.34; 95% confidence interval [CI] 1.09–1.65; $P<.006$). Additionally, development of AF after randomization was not affected by spironolactone but did significantly increase the incidence of the primary outcome (HR 2.32; 95% CI 1.59–3.40; $P<.0001$).[18]

This adverse prognostic prediction of AF with HF-pEF was also suggested by a retrospective study of 1744 HF-pEF patients from the Cleveland Clinic who underwent cardiopulmonary exercise testing (which included 239 with AF and HF-pEF). Peak $Vo_2$ and peak blood pressure was significantly lower in those with AF and HF-pEF than in those with HF-pEF alone (peak $Vo_2$ 18.5 ± 6.2 versus 20.3 ± 7.1 mL/kg per minute; $P<.0001$)

Moreover, AF was associated with higher total mortality over the follow-up period of the study.[19]

## STROKE PROPHYLAXIS

HF increases stroke and systemic embolism risk in AF via various mechanisms, with its risk being enough to justify inclusion in the most commonly used AF embolic risk score, the CHADS-VASc score. Congestive HF is assigned 1 point and as a result, therapeutic anticoagulation is recommended for any HF patient with AF (as males with a score ≥1 and females with a score ≥2 are recommended to be anticoagulated).[20]

Whether AF with HF-pEF or AF with HF-rEF has any individual impact on stroke risk has been assessed using several statistical methods. A prospective study of 1350 HF patients of important clinical outcomes in HF-pEF versus HF-rEF patients reported crude annual stroke and systemic embolism rates of 3.9% versus 2.7%, respectively, ($P = .47$). Age ≥75 years and B-type natriuretic protein level greater than 341 pg/mL were independent predictors of stroke and systemic embolism, irrespective of LVEF.[21] This important issue was also addressed in an analysis of the ACTIVE trial in which AF patients with HF were treated with clopidogrel (not oral anticoagulation) and treated with irbesartan for prevention of vascular events. HF-pEF patients exhibited embolic risk similar to that in those with HF-rEF (4.3 versus 4.4% per 100-person years [HR 1.01; 95% CI 0.78–1.31]).[22]

There is a lack of data supporting either HF-pEF or HF-rEF as subgroups conveying greater individual thrombotic risk of the other. Therefore, HF of any class should warrant strong consideration of therapeutic anticoagulation when AF develops. Warfarin was historically the mainstay of anticoagulation in AF with reduction in ischemic stroke rates of 68%; however, several direct oral anticoagulants including rivaroxaban, apixaban, dabigatran, and edoxaban are now in widespread use.[23–26]

## RHYTHM OR RATE CONTROL: HF-rEF

In 2008, a landmark study assessed the impact of a rate or rhythm-control strategy on outcomes of AF in 4060 patients that included 26% of patients with an LVEF ≤35%. The rates of death, stroke, and worsening HF were not statistically different depending upon which strategy was used over the mean follow-up period of 37 months.[27]

If a rate-control strategy is used, there is a degree of controversy about β-blocker prognostic benefit in HF-rEF patients with AF. Several large studies of β-blocker therapy in HF-rEF have clearly established their fundamental role in HF-rEF management, supported in international HF guidelines.[6,28,29] However, data from the SENIORS study, a randomized controlled study of nebivolol in HF patients, found no significant impact of nebivolol on the primary outcome specifically in AF patients, in contrast to the beneficial impact on patients in sinus rhythm.[30] In addition, a recent meta-analysis included 11 randomized studies of HF patients whereby compared with placebo, β-blockers were not associated with a mortality reduction in the subgroup of 3063 patients with AF, which is in stark contrast to the benefits of β-blocker therapy overall in HF-rEF (HR 0.96; 95% CI 0.81–1.12; $P = .58$).[31] Criticisms of this meta-analysis included the fact that subgroup analysis was not prespecified in the studies included in the analysis and that diagnosis of AF was based on a single baseline ECG in some of the studies, potentially misclassifying some of the patients.

In contrast, a more recent substudy of 1376 patients enrolled in the AF-CHF (a randomized control study of AF patients with HF) found that β-blocker use was associated with reduced mortality (HR 0.721; 95% CI 0.549–0.945; $P = .0180$), but did not impact on hospitalization rate (HR 0.886; 95% CI 0.715–1.100; $P = .2232$).[32] In addition, a large Danish registry of HF patients (which included 39,741 patients with AF and HF) found that β-blocker usage in HF-rEF patients was a favorable strategy, with a lower all-cause mortality (HR 0.75; 95% CI 0.71–0.79) and fatal thromboembolic event (HR 0.87; 95% CI 0.74–1.02) rates compared with nonusers of β-blockers.[33]

If β-blockers are not used as the rate-controlling agent (when such a strategy is adopted in an AF-HF patient), there are significant challenges with other pharmacologic alternatives. Nondihydropyrodine calcium-channel blockers are avoided in HF patients because of their negative inotropic effects, and digoxin is less efficacious in achieving rate control as isolated therapy, and has important safety considerations about toxicity rates and possible increased mortality in HF patients.

Rhythm control of AF, either electrically or pharmacologically, should be attempted in HF patients, particularly following an initial presentation of AF with HF-rEF or HF-pEF. Although there are no significant large-scale randomized trials to support the early restoration of sinus rhythm in AF with HF, the new AF presentation may have a reversible precipitant and, in proportion, may not recur after restoration of sinus rhythm. Restoring sinus rhythm provides maintenance of atrial function and avoids other mechanistic pathways for worsening HF. Addressing the thrombotic risk in the timing of restoration of sinus rhythm is of significant clinical importance.

When rhythm-control pharmacologic options are used in HF with AF, pharmacologic options include amiodarone, sotalol, and dofetilide (although there is geographic variability in its availability). Amiodarone can be used in the acute setting intravenously to achieve chemical cardioversion, or as an adjunct to electrical cardioversion. The long-term use of amiodarone should be avoided when possible given its well-documented potential for hepatic, thyroid, and pulmonary toxicity.

Sotalol may be used as an antiarrhythmic in HF-pEF patients and cautiously in selected HF-rEF patients. The SWORD study of the D-Sotalol formulation was a randomized study of patients with reduced LVEF (either after a recent myocardial infarction with LVEF <40%, or symptomatic HF with a remote myocardial infarction). D-Sotalol was associated with an increase in mortality compared with placebo.[34] However, the current formulation of sotalol has a different ratio of the D- and I-isomers and it does not significantly impair myocardial contractility in most patients.[35] It has been estimated that clinically significant HF aggravation only occurs in 1.5% to 3% of HF patients treated with sotalol, with a greater risk in those with an LVEF of less than 30%.[36–38]

## RHYTHM OR RATE CONTROL: HF-pEF

No large study has addressed whether a rhythm-control or rate-control strategy confers a mortality benefit in HF-pEF. However, observational evidence does suggest that maintaining sinus rhythm when possible may have a beneficial impact on quality of life, functional status, and survival.[39,40]

If a rate-control strategy is elected, β-blockers or the nondihydropyridine calcium-channel blockers diltiazem and verapamil can be safely used for rate control. Digoxin has historically been used for additional ventricular rate control and may be useful in specific AF patients with HF for adjunctive therapy. Some large observational studies have reported increasing mortality with digoxin; however, this has not been an entirely consistent finding across large studies of AF patients.[41,42] The large HF study (DIG trial) of digoxin in its ancillary cohort with LVEF greater than 45% demonstrated a reduction in HF hospitalizations and overall hospitalizations, but did not affect mortality.[43] If digoxin is used as an adjunctive therapy, diligence is essential for elderly patients and those

with renal dysfunction to avoid toxicity. A pharmacologic rhythm-control strategy in HF-pEF may be attempted with sotalol (with less concern than in HF-rEF for precipitating a decompensation) or amiodarone.

## ATRIOVENTRICULAR NODE ABLATION AND PACEMAKER IMPLANTATION

In patients with poorly controlled ventricular rates with persistent symptomatic AF, an intervention using implantation of a pacing device followed by an atrioventricular (AV) node ablation has been studied. This strategy his limited evidence of benefit in HF-rEF, with no major studies in AF with HF-pEF. However, occasionally all pharmacologic therapy fails and such a treatment warrants consideration in a very small proportion of HF patients.

When sinus rhythm can be maintained, improvement in cardiac function, and restoration of AV and interventricular synchrony by using cardio-resynchronization therapy (CRT) has been shown to correlate with a lower incidence of AF.[44] However, AF occurrence in patients with HF who receive a CRT device results in significantly less benefit from CRT with a higher rate of nonresponders (35% with AF versus 27% without AF, $P = .001$).[45]

A CRT implantation strategy was studied in a randomized controlled study that assessed the outcomes of 443 patients undergoing AV node ablation with CRT implantation, compared with 895 patients treated with medical rate control and 6046 patients in sinus rhythm. On multivariable analysis, AF and AV node ablation had a total mortality (HR 0.93; 95% CI 0.74–1.67) and cardiac mortality (HR 0.88; 95% CI 0.66–1.17) similar to that of the sinus rhythm group who were managed with such a strategy.[46]

Further studies are required to clarify this important issue in patients with chronic AF with wide QRS duration who have either HF-rEF or HF-pEF to determine whether there is any long-term clinical and mortality benefit to be derived from AV node ablation and pacing.

A direct comparison of catheter ablation with AV node ablation and biventricular pacing occurred in a prospective, multicenter clinical trial (PABA-CHF). This randomized study consisted of 81 AF patients with HF-rEF who had an LVEF of less than 40%. Catheter ablation resulted in a significant improvement in the primary end point at 6 months (Minnesota Living with Heart Failure Questionnaire Score), compared with AV node ablation and biventricular pacing. Catheter ablation was also associated with small benefits in measured 6-minute walk distance and LVEF.[47]

## CATHETER ABLATION IN HF-rEF

The benefit of catheter ablation in AF with HF when adopting a rhythm-control strategy was assessed in the multicenter ATTAC study. This randomized trial compared catheter ablation with amiodarone therapy in 203 patients who possessed HF-rEF (LVEF <40%), persisting AF, and New York Heart Association (NYHA) class II–III symptoms. At 24 months, 70% (95% CI 60%–78%), of the patients assigned to catheter ablation had AF-free survival versus 34% (95% CI 25%–44%; log-rank $P<.001$) in the control group. There were also benefits found in secondary end points of unplanned hospitalizations, overall mortality, and Minnesota Living with Heart Failure Questionnaire score.[48]

In the last 12 months, increasing evidence has emerged regarding the effectiveness of a rhythm-control strategy achieved via catheter ablation in patients with HF-rEF and AF. The CASTLE-HF study, a multicenter randomized control study, enrolled 397 patients across 31 centers with AF (either paroxysmal or permanent) and LVEF $\leq$35% (of any etiology). The primary end point was a composite of all-cause mortality and HF-related hospitalization. Randomization to catheter ablation resulted in reduction in the incidence of the primary end point, which occurred in 51 patients (28.5%), compared with 82 patients (44.6%) in the control group (HR 0.62; 95% CI 0.34–0.87; $P = .006$). This represented a risk reduction of 38% of the primary endpoint. AF burden was 25% in the catheter ablation group, compared with 60% in the medical therapy group.[49]

Further evidence of the benefit of catheter ablation was found in the CAMERA-MRI study, which was a randomized study assessing the prognostic value of myocardial fibrosis as assessed on post-gadolinium imaging to predict the outcome of catheter ablation in patients with AF combined with HF-rEF. In this study, 66 patients with nonischemic cardiomyopathy were randomized to catheter ablation of medical rate control. Catheter ablation was found to improve LVEF by 18% $\pm$ 13%, compared with medically treated patients who improved 4.4% $\pm$ 13% ($P<.0001$). The absence of late gadolinium enhancement predicted greater improvements in absolute LVEF (10.7%; $P = .0069$) and normalization at 6 months (73% versus 29%; $P = .0093$).[50]

Finally, a meta-analysis that included data from 7 studies and 856 HF-rEF patients found that catheter ablation was associated with decreased all-cause mortality, improved ejection fraction, and freedom of AF compared with medical treatment. There was no significant difference in the complication rates comparing catheter ablation with medical treatment.[51]

## CATHETER ABLATION IN HF-pEF

In contrast to HF-rEF, there is a paucity of well-designed large clinical studies assessing the effectiveness of catheter ablation for AF in patients specifically with HF-pEF. Part of the challenge of such a study is the design, given the heterogeneity of HF-pEF patients. However, a single-arm study of 74 patients with HF-pEF who underwent catheter ablation found reasonable success rates of 73% freedom from AF at 34 $\pm$ 16 months of follow-up. Maintenance of sinus rhythm was associated with echocardiographic improvement. However, many patients required multiple procedures as well as pharmaceutically assisted rhythm control after the procedure.[52]

Some further evidence supporting catheter ablation as a therapy in HF-pEF was demonstrated in a retrospective study of AF ablation in 230 HF patients (of which 57.8% had HF-pEF). Analysis of success and outcomes was reported with a comparison of HF-pEF versus HF-rEF diagnosis recorded at baseline. The procedural risks and procedural times were similar between the 2 groups. Freedom from recurrent atrial arrhythmia was not significantly different in HFpEF versus HFrEF patients (33.9% versus 32.6%; adjusted HR 1.47; 95% CI 0.72–3.01). There were also similar improvements in NYHA functional class (−0.32 versus −0.19; $P = .135$) after ablation.[53]

HF-pEF remains a large clinical challenge with a lack of proven prognostic pharmacotherapies, complex pathophysiology, and variable clinical presentation. AF with HF-pEF indicates an advanced phenotype. Whether successful catheter ablation can improve symptoms and mortality in this group is an area of desperately required research.

## LIFESTYLE MANAGEMENT AND INTEGRATED CARE IN HEART FAILURE WITH ATRIAL FIBRILLATION

Regardless of LVEF, aggressive management of lifestyle risk factors and comorbidities is paramount to achieving improved outcomes in AF with HF. Obesity, hypertension, and obstructive sleep apnea are important comorbidities of both HF-rEF and HF-pEF. Obesity is a major risk factor for development of AF, increases the risk of HF development, and has an evolving identifiable HF-pEF phenotype.[54,55] The benefits and safety of exercise in HF (across LVEFs) are well established from the HF-ACTION study, which demonstrated improvements following participation in an exercise program in functional capacity, peak oxygen consumption, and cardiopulmonary exercise duration.[56] In addition, exercise benefits in HF are also supported by a recent trial of intentional weight loss and exercise in obese elderly patients with HF-PEF that demonstrated a significant improvement in exercise capacity as measured by peak oxygen consumption.[57] Previous studies in AF have also demonstrated the impact of weight loss and lifestyle intervention on outcomes.[58]

The recently published RACE 3 study provided strong evidence of the role of targeted therapy in AF management. This was a randomized study that targeted risk factors and comorbidities in an AF population of 245 patients. The intervention (which occurred in 119 patients) consisted of pharmacotherapy including prescription of mineralocorticoid receptor antagonists, statins, angiotensin-converting enzyme inhibitors and/or receptor blockers, and involvement in a cardiac rehabilitation program consisting of physical activity, dietary restriction, and counseling. The intervention group had higher rate of sinus rhythm at 1 year (75%) compared with the control group (63%) (odds ratio 1.765; lower limit of 95% CI 1.021; $P = .042$).[59]

An integrated approach that includes cardiologists (both an electrophysiologist and HF physician) and specialized AF and HF nurses provides a clinical networking framework that addresses individual patient understanding, psychological support, and important lifestyle factors to optimize AF and HF outcomes.

## SUMMARY

AF and HF are major international health care challenges that commonly occur together. Assessment of LV systolic function, which is primarily performed with echocardiography, is a vital aspect in the evaluation of the newly presenting AF patient. HF-rEF and HF-pEF are substantially growing in their incidence and AF commonly occurs in both syndromes. Some aspects of the pivotal clinical management of AF have similarities with that of HF-pEF and HF-rEF. Restoration of sinus rhythm from AF in the HF patient (regardless of whether HF-rEF or HF-pEF) is favorable if this can be achieved and maintained. However, a significant number of HF patients will develop recurrent paroxysmal AF and permanent AF. For such patients, whether to adopt a rate-control or rhythm-control strategy is a key decision. There are minimal differences in AF with HF-pEF and HF-rEF with regard to thromboembolic risk and the strong indication for therapeutic anticoagulation. Lifestyle and risk factor management are essential in both

groups of HF, particularly when significant risk factors such as obesity are present. A growing body of evidence supports catheter ablation in HF-rEF patients with AF who are well selected for this procedure. A small number of studies has demonstrated safety of catheter ablation in HF-pEF, although further data are needed from this group in a well-designed clinical trial.

## REFERENCES

1. Sartipy U, Dahlstrom U, Fu M, et al. Atrial fibrillation in heart failure with preserved, mid-range, and reduced ejection fraction. JACC Heart Fail 2017; 5(8):565–74.
2. Santhanakrishnan R, Wang N, Larson MG, et al. Atrial fibrillation begets heart failure and vice versa: temporal associations and differences in preserved vs. reduced ejection fraction. Circulation 2016; 133(5):484–92.
3. Miyasaka Y, Barnes ME, Gersh BJ, et al. Secular trends in incidence of atrial fibrillation in Olmsted County, Minnesota, 1980 to 2000, and implications on the projections for future prevalence. Circulation 2006;114(2):119–25.
4. Zakeri R, Chamberlain AM, Roger VL, et al. Temporal relationship and prognostic significance of atrial fibrillation in heart failure patients with preserved ejection fraction: a community-based study. Circulation 2013;128(10):1085–93.
5. Xu B, Klein AL. Utility of echocardiography in heart failure with preserved ejection fraction. J Card Fail 2018;24(6):397–403.
6. Ponikowski P, Voors AA, Anker SD, et al. 2016 ESC guidelines for the diagnosis and treatment of acute and chronic heart failure: the Task Force for the diagnosis and treatment of acute and chronic heart failure of the European Society of Cardiology (ESC) developed with the special contribution of the Heart Failure Association (HFA) of the ESC. Eur Heart J 2016;37(27):2129–200.
7. Meluzin J, Starek Z, Kulik T, et al. Prevalence and predictors of early heart failure with preserved ejection fraction in patients with paroxysmal atrial fibrillation. J Card Fail 2017;23(7):558–62.
8. Reddy YNV, Olson TP, Obokata M, et al. Hemodynamic correlates and diagnostic role of cardiopulmonary exercise testing in heart failure with preserved ejection fraction. JACC Heart Fail 2018; 6(8):665–75.
9. Gopinathannair R, Etheridge SP, Marchlinski FE, et al. Arrhythmia-induced cardiomyopathies: mechanisms, recognition, and management. J Am Coll Cardiol 2015;66(15):1714–28.
10. Blume GG, McLeod CJ, Barnes ME, et al. Left atrial function: physiology, assessment, and clinical implications. Eur J Echocardiogr 2011;12(6):421–30.

11. Shinbane JS, Wood MA, Jensen DN, et al. Tachy-cardia-induced cardiomyopathy: a review of animal models and clinical studies. J Am Coll Cardiol 1997;29(4):709–15.

12. Tuinenburg AE, Van Veldhuisen DJ, Boomsma F, et al. Comparison of plasma neurohormones in congestive heart failure patients with atrial fibrillation versus patients with sinus rhythm. Am J Cardiol 1998;81(10):1207–10.

13. Ling LH, Kistler PM, Kalman JM, et al. Comorbidity of atrial fibrillation and heart failure. Nat Rev Cardiol 2016;13(3):131–47.

14. Li D, Fareh S, Leung TK, et al. Promotion of atrial fibrillation by heart failure in dogs: atrial remodeling of a different sort. Circulation 1999;100(1):87–95.

15. Sridhar A, Nishijima Y, Terentyev D, et al. Chronic heart failure and the substrate for atrial fibrillation. Cardiovasc Res 2009;84(2):227–36.

16. Leong DP, Dokainish H. Left atrial volume and function in patients with atrial fibrillation. Curr Opin Cardiol 2014;29(5):437–44.

17. Vizzardi E, Curnis A, Latini MG, et al. Risk factors for atrial fibrillation recurrence: a literature review. J Cardiovasc Med (Hagerstown) 2014;15(3):235–53.

18. Cikes M, Claggett B, Shah AM, et al. Atrial fibrillation in heart failure with preserved ejection fraction: the TOPCAT trial. JACC Heart Fail 2018;6(8):689–97.

19. Elshazly MB, Senn T, Wu Y, et al. Impact of atrial fibrillation on exercise capacity and mortality in heart failure with preserved ejection fraction: insights from cardiopulmonary stress testing. J Am Heart Assoc 2017;6(11) [pii:e006662].

20. Agarwal M, Apostolakis S, Lane DA, et al. The impact of heart failure and left ventricular dysfunction in predicting stroke, thromboembolism, and mortality in atrial fibrillation patients: a systematic review. Clin Ther 2014;36(9):1135–44.

21. Sobue Y, Watanabe E, Lip GYH, et al. Thromboembolisms in atrial fibrillation and heart failure patients with a preserved ejection fraction (HFpEF) compared to those with a reduced ejection fraction (HFrEF). Heart Vessels 2018;33(4):403–12.

22. Sandhu RK, Hohnloser SH, Pfeffer MA, et al. Relationship between degree of left ventricular dysfunction, symptom status, and risk of embolic events in patients with atrial fibrillation and heart failure. Stroke 2015;46(3):667–72.

23. Hart RG, Sherman DG, Easton JD. Atrial fibrillation and stroke. Stroke 1984;15(2):387–8.

24. Connolly SJ, Ezekowitz MD, Yusuf S, et al. Dabigatran versus warfarin in patients with atrial fibrillation. N Engl J Med 2009;361(12):1139–51.

25. Granger CB, Alexander JH, McMurray JJ, et al. Apixaban versus warfarin in patients with atrial fibrillation. N Engl J Med 2011;365(11):981–92.

26. Patel MR, Mahaffey KW, Garg J, et al. Rivaroxaban versus warfarin in nonvalvular atrial fibrillation. N Engl J Med 2011;365(10):883–91.

27. Roy D, Talajic M, Nattel S, et al. Rhythm control versus rate control for atrial fibrillation and heart failure. N Engl J Med 2008;358(25):2667–77.

28. Poole-Wilson PA, Swedberg K, Cleland JG, et al. Comparison of carvedilol and metoprolol on clinical outcomes in patients with chronic heart failure in the Carvedilol or Metoprolol European Trial (COMET): randomised controlled trial. Lancet 2003;362(9377):7–13.

29. Packer M, Fowler MB, Roecker EB, et al. Effect of carvedilol on the morbidity of patients with severe chronic heart failure: results of the carvedilol prospective randomized cumulative survival (CO-PERNICUS) study. Circulation 2002;106(17):2194–9.

30. Mulder BA, van Veldhuisen DJ, Crijns HJ, et al. Effect of nebivolol on outcome in elderly patients with heart failure and atrial fibrillation: insights from SENIORS. Eur J Heart Fail 2012;14(10):1171–8.

31. Kotecha D, Flather MD, Altman DG, et al. Heart rate and rhythm and the benefit of beta-blockers in patients with heart failure. J Am Coll Cardiol 2017;69(24):2885–96.

32. Cadrin-Tourigny J, Shohoudi A, Roy D, et al. Decreased mortality with beta-blockers in patients with heart failure and coexisting atrial fibrillation: an AF-CHF substudy. JACC Heart Fail 2017;5(2):99–106.

33. Nielsen PB, Larsen TB, Gorst-Rasmussen A, et al. Beta-blockers in atrial fibrillation patients with or without heart failure: association with mortality in a nationwide cohort study. Circ Heart Fail 2016;9(2):e002597.

34. Waldo AL, Camm AJ, deRuyter H, et al. Effect of d-sotalol on mortality in patients with left ventricular dysfunction after recent and remote myocardial infarction. The SWORD Investigators. Survival with Oral d-Sotalol. Lancet 1996;348(9019):7–12.

35. Hohnloser SH, Woosley RL. Sotalol. N Engl J Med 1994;331(1):31–8.

36. Kehoe RF, Zheutlin TA, Dunnington CS, et al. Safety and efficacy of sotalol in patients with drug-refractory sustained ventricular tachyarrhythmias. Am J Cardiol 1990;65(2):58A–64A [discussion: 65A–6A].

37. Soyka LF, Wirtz C, Spangenberg RB. Clinical safety profile of sotalol in patients with arrhythmias. Am J Cardiol 1990;65(2):74A–81A [discussion: 82A–3A].

38. Anderson JL, Prystowsky EN. Sotalol: an important new antiarrhythmic. Am Heart J 1999;137(3):388–409.

39. Corley SD, Epstein AE, DiMarco JP, et al. Relationships between sinus rhythm, treatment, and survival in the atrial fibrillation follow-up investigation of

rhythm management (AFFIRM) study. Circulation 2004;109(12):1509–13.

40. Kosior DA, Szulc M, Rosiak M, et al. Functional status with rhythm versus rate control strategies for persistent atrial fibrillation. Pol Arch Intern Med 2018;128(11):658–66.

41. Gheorghiade M, Fonarow GC, van Veldhuisen DJ, et al. Lack of evidence of increased mortality among patients with atrial fibrillation taking digoxin: findings from post hoc propensity-matched analysis of the AFFIRM trial. Eur Heart J 2013;34(20):1489–97.

42. Turakhia MP, Santangeli P, Winkelmayer WC, et al. Increased mortality associated with digoxin in contemporary patients with atrial fibrillation: findings from the TREAT-AF study. J Am Coll Cardiol 2014; 64(7):660–8.

43. Digitalis Investigation Group. The effect of digoxin on mortality and morbidity in patients with heart failure. N Engl J Med 1997;336(8):525–33.

44. Fung JW, Yip GW, Yu CM. Does atrial fibrillation preclude biventricular pacing? Heart 2008;94(7):826–7.

45. Wilton SB, Leung AA, Ghali WA, et al. Outcomes of cardiac resynchronization therapy in patients with versus those without atrial fibrillation: a systematic review and meta-analysis. Heart Rhythm 2011;8(7): 1088–94.

46. Gasparini M, Leclercq C, Lunati M, et al. Cardiac resynchronization therapy in patients with atrial fibrillation: the CERTIFY study (cardiac resynchronization therapy in atrial fibrillation patients multinational registry). JACC Heart Fail 2013;1(6):500–7.

47. Khan MN, Jais P, Cummings J, et al. Pulmonary-vein isolation for atrial fibrillation in patients with heart failure. N Engl J Med 2008;359(17):1778–85.

48. Di Biase L, Mohanty P, Mohanty S, et al. Ablation versus amiodarone for treatment of persistent atrial fibrillation in patients with congestive heart failure and an implanted device: results from the AATAC multicenter randomized trial. Circulation 2016; 133(17):1637–44.

49. Marrouche NF, Brachmann J, Andresen D, et al. Catheter ablation for atrial fibrillation with heart failure. N Engl J Med 2018;378(5):417–27.

50. Prabhu S, Taylor AJ, Costello BT, et al. Catheter ablation versus medical rate control in atrial fibrillation and systolic dysfunction: the CAMERA-MRI Study. J Am Coll Cardiol 2017;70(16): 1949–61.

51. Briceno DF, Markman TM, Lupercio F, et al. Catheter ablation versus conventional treatment of atrial fibrillation in patients with heart failure with reduced ejection fraction: a systematic review and meta-analysis of randomized controlled trials. J Interv Card Electrophysiol 2018;53(1):19–29.

52. Machino-Ohtsuka T, Seo Y, Ishizu T, et al. Efficacy, safety, and outcomes of catheter ablation of atrial fibrillation in patients with heart failure with preserved ejection fraction. J Am Coll Cardiol 2013; 62(20):1857–65.

53. Black-Maier E, Ren X, Steinberg BA, et al. Catheter ablation of atrial fibrillation in patients with heart failure and preserved ejection fraction. Heart Rhythm 2018;15(5):651–7.

54. Kitzman DW, Lam CSP. Obese heart failure with preserved ejection fraction phenotype: from pariah to central player. Circulation 2017;136(1):20–3.

55. Kenchaiah S, Evans JC, Levy D, et al. Obesity and the risk of heart failure. N Engl J Med 2002;347(5): 305–13.

56. O'Connor CM, Whellan DJ, Lee KL, et al. Efficacy and safety of exercise training in patients with chronic heart failure: HF-ACTION randomized controlled trial. JAMA 2009;301(14):1439–50.

57. Kitzman DW, Brubaker P, Morgan T, et al. Effect of caloric restriction or aerobic exercise training on peak oxygen consumption and quality of life in obese older patients with heart failure with preserved ejection fraction: a randomized clinical trial. JAMA 2016;315(1):36–46.

58. Pathak RK, Middeldorp ME, Meredith M, et al. Long-term effect of goal-directed weight management in an atrial fibrillation cohort: a long-term follow-up study (LEGACY). J Am Coll Cardiol 2015;65(20): 2159–69.

59. Rienstra M, Hobbelt AH, Alings M, et al. Targeted therapy of underlying conditions improves sinus rhythm maintenance in patients with persistent atrial fibrillation: results of the RACE 3 trial. Eur Heart J 2018;39(32):2987–96.

# Randomized Clinical Trials of Catheter Ablation of Atrial Fibrillation in Congestive Heart Failure
## Knowns and Unmet Needs

Maria Terricabras, MD[a],
Jonathan P. Piccini Sr, MD, MHS, FHRS[b],
Atul Verma, MD, FRCPC, FHRS[a],*

### KEYWORDS

- Atrial fibrillation • Catheter ablation • Heart failure • Outcomes • Randomized clinical trial

### KEY POINTS

- Rhythm control strategy with antiarrhythmic drugs failed to demonstrate benefit in patients with heart failure and reduced ejection fraction (HFrEF).
- Catheter ablation is an effective strategy for maintenance of sinus rhythm in patients with HFrEF.
- Randomized clinical trials have demonstrated the potential benefit of catheter ablation in patients with HF, including improvement in quality of life, symptoms, and left ventricular function.
- Emerging evidence from randomized clinical trials suggests that catheter ablation of atrial fibrillation may improve cardiovascular outcomes in patients with HFrEF, such as hospitalization and cardiovascular death.

## INTRODUCTION

Atrial fibrillation (AF) increases morbidity and mortality in patients with heart failure and reduced ejection fraction (HFrEF). These 2 conditions frequently coexist and impact reciprocally on each other. The interaction between these 2 conditions is complex, and each can promote the occurrence of the other. Furthermore, many antiarrhythmic medications used to treat AF are contraindicated in the presence of structural heart disease and HFrEF, and other medications, like beta-blockers, may not be as effective in HFrEF patients with AF.[1] Consequently, the question of how to optimally treat AF in heart failure (HF) patients remains a major challenge for clinicians.[2,3]

## CLINICAL TRIALS OF ANTIARRHYTHMIC DRUG TREATMENT

The first seminal study examining this challenge was the Atrial Fibrillation and Congestive Heart Failure (AF-CHF) trial. The trial tested the hypothesis that maintaining sinus rhythm with a rhythm control

Disclosure Statement: M. Terricabras declares no conflicts of interest. J.P. Piccini receives funding for clinical research from Abbott, ARCA Biopharma, Boston Scientific, Gilead, Janssen Pharmaceuticals, and NHLBI and serves as a consultant to Abbott, Allergan, ARCA Biopharma, Bayer, Biotronik, GSK, Johnson & Johnson, Medtronic, Motif Bio, Sanofi, and Phillips. A. Verma reports grants from Bayer, Biosense Webster, and Medtronic.
a Southlake Regional Health Centre, University of Toronto, Suite 602, 581 Davis Drive, Newmarket, Ontario L3Y 2P6, Canada; b Duke Center for Atrial Fibrillation, Duke University Medical Center, Duke Clinical Research Institute, DUMC #3115, Durham, NC 27705, USA
* Corresponding author.
E-mail address: atul.verma@utoronto.ca

Cardiol Clin 37 (2019) 167–176
https://doi.org/10.1016/j.ccl.2019.01.003
0733-8651/19/

strategy would change the natural history of both conditions in patients with HFrEF and prove superior to a strategy of rate control alone. Despite expectations for improved outcomes with pharmacologic rhythm control, the rhythm control arm (predominantly amiodarone) failed to improve all-cause survival compared with rate control. In fact, AF-CHF demonstrated that rhythm control was associated with an increased risk of all-cause hospitalization. Another study of antiarrhythmic drug (AAD) treatment in patients with HFrEF, the Danish Investigators Of Arrhythmia And Mortality On Dofetilde Congestive Heart Failure (DIAMOND CHF) trial, randomized 1018 patients with New York Heart Association (NYHA) class III–IV HF and left ventricular ejection fraction (LVEF) less than 35% to placebo or the class III AAD dofetilide. Although dofetilide was associated with a lower risk of HF hospitalization, there was no evidence of improved survival compared with placebo. Given the lack of benefit with rhythm control in AF-CHF and DIAMOND-CHF, it is not surprising, then, that most international guidelines recommend rate control as the first-line therapy for AF in patients with HFrEF. These guidelines also recommended rhythm control only for those patients with ongoing symptoms secondary to AF despite rate control.[4,5]

Although early trials failed to demonstrate superiority of a rhythm control strategy in AF with HFrEF, the hypothesis that aggressive and effective maintenance of sinus rhythm should improve outcomes in patients with HFrEF remains enticing. There are several reasons that AAD therapy may not improve outcomes, including the limited efficacy of these drugs to maintain sinus rhythm. The absolute increase in the proportion of patients in sinus rhythm with AAD treatment was only +28% in DIAMOND CHF and +32% in AF-CHF. The other possibility is that the beneficial effects of maintaining sinus rhythm with AADs are abrogated by the occurrence of adverse events, and in the case of amiodarone, end organ toxicities. A rhythm control intervention that is more effective, durable, and safer than AAD therapy offers the theoretic benefit of improved cardiovascular outcomes that are otherwise unrealized with current drug treatment.

Catheter ablation (CA) has emerged as an important alternative to AAD for maintaining sinus rhythm in patients with paroxysmal and persistent forms of AF. Numerous studies have shown that ablation is superior to AAD for achieving sinus rhythm both for patients who are refractory to drugs or for first-line therapy, but none of these trials focused on patients with ventricular dysfunction.[6–8] Large registries have also shown that CA of AF is a safe procedure with a low rate of major complications.[9,10] As such, CA may yield a long-

term safety advantage given the potential deleterious effects of long-term AAD therapy,[4,11] especially in patients with HFrEF and limited AAD options (dofetilide or amiodarone).[12] In addition to improved maintenance of sinus rhythm, observational studies and randomized trials have shown improvement in postablation ejection fraction (EF), quality of life (QoL), and functional capacity in the AF and HFrEF population.[13,14]

Although the rationale for using CA to treat AF in the HFrEF population may seem promising, the efficacy and safety of this procedure in patients with HFrEF remain uncertain. In this article, the authors review the available randomized data available to compare CA to medical therapy alone in the AF and HF population as well as the unmet needs in this challenging population.

## RANDOMIZED TRIALS: SURROGATE ENDPOINTS: PROOF OF CONCEPT

There have been a few, very small randomized trials in which surrogate endpoints, such as reverse ventricular remodeling or peak oxygen consumption, have been used to demonstrate proof of concept, that CA of AF might benefit patients with HFrEF (**Table 1**).

### PABA-CHF: Pulmonary-vein Isolation for Atrial Fibrillation in Patients with Heart Failure

This study published in 2008 was the first randomized trial to compare AF ablation with rate control in patients with EF of 40% or less. The investigators randomized 81 patients with symptomatic AF despite the use of AAD to receive a pulmonary vein isolation (PVI) procedure or an atrioventricular node ablation with biventricular pacing. All the patients included had NYHA class II–III symptoms, were prescribed optimal medical treatment of HF, and had no previous history of surgical or catheter AF ablation. The primary endpoints in PABA-CHF were change in LVEF, distance on the 6-minute walk test (6MWT), and improvement in the QoL Minnesota Living with Heart Failure (MLWHF) questionnaire at 6-month follow-up. PVI was required, and additional linear ablation or ablation of complex fractionated atrial electrograms (CFAE) was left to operator discretion. The results following ablation were good: 71% of the patients in the PVI arm were free from AF (including repeat procedures) off AAD (88% with AAD), but only half of the patients were in persistent AF (49% paroxysmal and 51% persistent). There was improvement in all endpoints in both groups but significantly better improvement in the ablation arm, including LVEF (35% ± 9% vs 28% ± 6%, $P<.001$), 6-minute walking distance

**Table 1**
**Summary of the randomized clinical trials**

| Study, y | Sample Size (CA) | Comparison Group | Population Characteristics | Primary Endpoint | Follow-Up (mo) | Success Rate CA (≥1 Procedure) (%) | Ablation Strategy | Complications (per Patient) (%) |
|---|---|---|---|---|---|---|---|---|
| Khan et al,[15] 2008 PABA-CHF | 81 (41) | AV nodal ablation + BiV pacing | LVEF <40% NYHA II or III Persistent or paroxysmal AF | Composite of EF, 6MWT, and MLWHF score | 6 | 71 | PVI ± lines ± CFAE | 12.2 |
| MacDonald et al,[19] 2011 | 41 (22) | Rate control | LVEF <35% NYHA II-IV Persistent AF | Improvement in LVEF measured by MRI[a] | 6 | 50 | PVI ± lines ± CFAE | 27.3 MAE 14.8 |
| Jones et al,[16] 2013 ARC-HF | 52 (26) | Rate control | LVEF <35% NYHA II-IV Persistent AF | Change in peak oxygen consumption | 12 | 92 | PVI + roof and mitral lines + CTI + CFAE | 15.4 MAE 3.8 |
| Hunter et al,[17] 2014 CAMTAF | 50 (26) | Rate control | LVEF <50% NYHA II-IV Persistent AF | Improvement in LVEF (echo) | 6 (1 y CA) | 81 (6 mo) 73 (1 y) | PVI + CFAE ± roof line and mitral line | MAE 7.7 |
| Di Biase et al,[20] 2016 AATAC | 203 (102) | Amiodarone | LVEF <40%, NYHA II-III ICD or CRT-D Persistent AF | Recurrence of AF | 24 | 70 | PVI + posterior wall + CFAE + non-PV triggers (78%) | 2.9 |
| Prabhu et al,[18] 2017 CAMERA-MRI | 68 (33) | Rate control | LVEF <45% (CMR) NYHA II-IV Persistent AF No CAD or other cause for LV dysfunction | Change in LVEF (MRI) | 6 | 56 | PVI + posterior wall | 6.1 |
| Marrouche et al,[21] 2018 CASTLE-AF | 363 (179) | Medical therapy (rate or rhythm) | LVEF <35%, Paroxysmal or persistent AF NYHA II-IV ICD or CRT-D | Composite of death for any cause or worsening HF | 37.8 | 63 | PVI | 8.4 |

*Abbreviation:* MAE, major adverse events.
[a] No significant difference found between both arms.

(340 ± 49 m vs 297 ± 36 m, P<.001), and MLWHF scores (60 ± 8 vs 82 ± 14, P<.001).[15]

### ARC-HF: A Randomized Trial to Assess Catheter Ablation Versus Rate Control in the Management of Persistent Atrial Fibrillation in Heart Failure

Jones and colleagues[16] conducted a similar trial whereby 52 subjects were randomized to receive CA or optimal rate control therapy. The inclusion criteria were simple: persistent AF, symptomatic HF symptoms despite optimal medical treatment, and LVEF less than 35%. The primary endpoint was change in peak oxygen consumption at 12-month follow-up, and secondary endpoints included improvement in QoL, reduction in brain natriuretic peptide (BNP) levels, change in 6MWT, and LVEF. The success rate of AF ablation after a single procedure and off AAD in this study was 72% (multiprocedure 92%). The procedure comprised PVI, linear ablation, and elimination of left atrial CFAEs. Patients in the ablation arm experienced an increase in peak $Vo_2$ +2.13 (95% confidence interval [CI] −0.10 to +4.36) mL/kg/min compared with a decrease in the medical therapy arm −0.94 (95% CI −2.21 to +0.32) mL/kg/min (P = .018). There was also a significant improvement in the QoL at 12 months (P = .019) and a significant decrease in the BNP levels (P = .045) in the ablation arm compared with the medical therapy arm. However, there was no significant improvement in 6MWT. Finally, EF showed a trend toward improvement in the ablation arm compared with rate control, but it was nonsignificant (P = .055).

### CAMTAF Trial: A Randomized Controlled Trial of Catheter Ablation Versus Medical Treatment of Atrial Fibrillation in Heart Failure

Hunter and colleagues[17] also conducted a relatively small trial that randomized 50 patients in a 1:1 fashion to receive CA versus medical therapy alone with a rate control strategy. Eligible patients had to be in persistent AF and have NYHA class II–IV symptoms, and left ventricular (LV) systolic dysfunction with LVEF less than 50%. Despite the inclusion criteria, the mean LVEF in the ablation group was 31.8% versus 33.7% in the rate control group, comparable to the above described studies. The ablation procedure included PVI and ablation of CFAEs in the left and right atria, and if the patients did not restore sinus rhythm, additional lines were performed on the roof and mitral isthmus. Surprisingly, the success rate with a single procedure was only 38%. Fourteen patients (54%) underwent a second procedure, and 3 required a third procedure (12%). The success

rates after the last procedure without AAD was 81% at 6 months and 73% at 12 months. The primary endpoint was the change in LVEF from baseline to 6 months, which was significantly better in the ablation arm (+8.1% vs −3,6%, P<.001). Secondary endpoints also supported the benefit of CA with an increase in $Vo_{2max}$, lower BNP determination, and improvement in symptoms and QoL. Taken together, these findings reinforced the positive results from ARC-HF and PABA-CHF.

### CAMERA-MRI: Catheter Ablation Versus Medical Rate Control in Atrial Fibrillation and Systolic Dysfunction

This clinical trial sought to assess the outcomes of AF ablation compared with rate control in patients with LV dysfunction in whom the cause of the cardiomyopathy was unexplained beyond the presence of AF. All the previously described studies included a wide variety of patients with cardiomyopathy of varied causes, most of which were ischemic cardiomyopathy. In CAMERA, the inclusion criteria were NYHA class II–IV symptoms, persistent AF, LVEF less than 45%, absence of significant coronary artery disease, or other causes of LV dysfunction. PVI and posterior wall isolation were required in all subjects in the ablation arm. The primary endpoint was a change in LVEF after 6-month follow-up. A significant increase was reported in both groups but was superior in the ablation group (18.3% vs 4.4%, P≤.0001). In fact, 58% of the patients in the ablation arm had complete normalization of the LVEF. The investigators reported a single procedure success rate of 56% off AAD and 75% on AAD. Regarding the secondary endpoints assessed, there was a significant reduction of the LV end systolic volume in the ablation arm compared with the medical arm (−24 ± 24 mL/m$^2$ vs −8.0 ± 20 mL/m$^2$ P = .007), as well as the left atrium volume (−12 ± 13 mL/m$^2$ vs 1.7 ± 14 mL/m$^2$; P<.0001). BNP levels significantly decreased, and QoL was also significantly better in the ablation group. Another interesting finding was the relationship between the absence of ventricular late gadolinium enhancement and greater improvement in LVEF after the procedure. This study showed that for patients with so-called rate-related cardiomyopathy secondary to AF, rate control may not be sufficient for complete resolution of the cardiomyopathy. The medical therapy arm had appropriate rate control monitored by implantable loop recorder but did not experience the same improvement as the ablation arm. The results form CAMERA-MRI suggest that factors beyond tachycardic heart rates, such as irregular ventricular contractions, loss of atrial contraction, or activation of neurohormonal and profibrotic pathways, may play an important role in AF-related LV dysfunction.[18]

### Radiofrequency Ablation for Persistent Atrial Fibrillation in Patients with Advanced Heart Failure and Severe Left Ventricular Systolic Dysfunction

The one exception to the positive trials described above was that of MacDonald and colleagues.[19] They compared rhythm control with CA with rate control with medical therapy. All patients enrolled in this study had NYHA class II–IV symptoms despite optimal medical treatment, LVEF less than 35%, and persistent AF. Forty-one patients were included: 22 were randomized to receive CA and 19 were randomized to receive medical therapy. PVI was required in all patients and additional lines and CFAE in both the right and the left atrium when AF persisted after successful PVI. The follow-up was 6 months, and primary endpoint was change in LVEF measured by cardiac MRI. Secondary endpoints included improvement in QoL, in NT-pro-BNP level, and in 6MWD. Only 50% of the patients in the PVI group were in sinus rhythm after 6 months. Moreover, there was a 15% rate of major complications in the ablation group. Ablation did not significantly improve the LVEF measured by magnetic resonance compared with the medical therapy group (+4.5% ± 11.1% vs +2.8% ± 6.7%, $P = .6$), and there was no difference in QoL, pro-BNP levels, nor 6MWD. The negative results may have been due to the lower success rate of AF ablation and the higher rate of complications. The population also had a higher proportion of patients with advanced HF (approximately 90% of the subjects had NYHA class III symptoms) and long-standing persistent AF. Therefore, although the cumulative results of these proof-of-concept trials support the idea that ablation may benefit patients with HFrEF and AF, the caveats are that the ablation procedure has to be effective with a low rate of complications and the HF population likely cannot be too far advanced.[19] CA may come too late in patients with advanced HF and end-stage atrial myopathy.

### RANDOMIZED TRIALS: "HARDER" ENDPOINTS: MOVING TOWARD BROADER CLINICAL APPLICATION

More recently, some larger trials have been performed that focused on cardiovascular outcomes, including HF hospitalization and all-cause mortality, in an attempt to provide evidence beyond "proof of concept" to support broader clinical application in patients with AF and HF (**Table 1**).

### AATAC Trial: Ablation Versus Amiodarone for Treatment of Persistent Atrial Fibrillation in Patients with Congestive Heart Failure and an implanted device

This larger study randomized 203 patients with persistent AF, dual-chamber implantable cardioverter defibrillators (ICD), or cardiac resynchronization therapy defibrillators, NYHA class II–III HF symptoms, and LV dysfunction (LVEF <40%) to either AF ablation (n = 102) or rhythm control with amiodarone (n = 101) with a 24-month follow-up. Although the primary endpoint was freedom from AF, secondary endpoints included hospitalization and mortality. In the ablation group, 78% of the subjects received an extensive ablation with PVI, posterior wall isolation, and ablation of CFAE and nonpulmonary vein (PV) triggers. With an average of 1.4 procedures, 70% of the subjects were free from recurrent AF in the ablation group compared with only 34% in the amiodarone group ($P \leq .001$). Notably, for the first time, this trial showed that ablation might have an impact on standard cardiovascular outcomes used in HF trials. Unplanned hospitalizations, for example, were significantly lower in the ablation group with a relative risk reduction (RRR) of 45% compared with amiodarone, with a number needed to treat (NNT) of 3.8 to avoid 1 unplanned hospitalization. All-cause mortality showed a significant 56% RRR with ablation. Finally, despite including patients with HF and reduced EF, the procedural complications were very low (2% vascular complications and 1% pericardial effusion).[20]

### CASTLE-AF: Catheter Ablation for Atrial Fibrillation with Heart Failure

Marrouche and colleagues[21] recently published the results of CASTLE-AF, the largest of all the AF ablation trials focused on patients with HFrEF. CASTLE-AF was a cardiovascular outcomes trial with a primary endpoint of death or HF hospitalization. The investigators randomized 363 patients with HFrEF to receive PVI ablation or medical therapy alone, which included both rate and rhythm control. All the subjects enrolled were in persistent or paroxysmal AF, had LVEF ≤35%, with at least NYHA class II symptoms, an ICD or implantable cardiac resynchronization therapy defibrillator (CRT-D) implant, and absence of response to AAD, unacceptable side effects or to patient refusal to take them. The risk of HF hospitalization or death over median follow-up of 38 months was lower in the ablation group compared with the medical group (28.5% vs 44.6%; $P = .006$). In secondary analysis, ablation was also associated with significantly lower all-cause mortality compared with medical therapy (13.4% vs 25%, $P = .01$), and cardiovascular death was reduced by approximately 50% with ablation (hazard ratio [HR] 0.49, 95% CI 0.29–0.84, $P = .009$). Cardiovascular hospitalization was also significantly reduced in the ablation group (35.8% vs 48.4%, $P = .04$). At the 60-month follow-up visit, 63% of patients were in sinus rhythm in the ablation group (average of 1.3 procedures per patient) versus 22% in the medical therapy group. The results from CASTLE-AF certainly generate a great deal of enthusiasm for ablation in patients with AF and HF, but a major caveat needs to be emphasized. The population included in CASTLE was carefully selected, of more than 3000 patients screened, only about 10% were selected for enrollment; these patients also needed to have failed or found unsuitable for AAD before inclusion. It is perhaps not surprising, then, that such a select group of individuals would have had such a dramatic reduction in both mortality and hospitalization with ablation compared with medical therapy. Needless to say, CASTLE provided the first indication that CA might play a clinically substantive role in altering the natural history of patients with HFrEF and AF.

## CABANA: Catheter Ablation vs Antiarrhythmic Drug Therapy for Atrial Fibrillation

Although CABANA was not a trial specifically designed to examine the role of AF ablation in patients with HF, about 15% of the 2204 patients enrolled (n = 337) had a history of congestive HF (CASTLE enrolled 363 patients). Not all of these patients had HFrEF because only about 10% of CABANA patients had a documented history of cardiomyopathy. Overall, CABANA did not demonstrate a significant difference between first-line ablation and medical therapy for the primary composite of death, disabling stroke, serious bleeding, or cardiac arrest by intention to treat. However, in the subgroup of patients with HF, there was a strong trend toward benefit of ablation (HR 0.61, 95% CI 0.35–1.08), which was statistically significant in the "per-protocol" or "as-treated" analysis (HR 0.51, 95% CI 0.28–0.91). At the time of writing this article, the final results of CABANA are as yet unpublished, as are the results of the HF subgroup. However, these preliminary results certainly offer some insights, and for the first time, offer some possibility of improvement in patients with AF and heart failure with preserved ejection fraction (HFpEF).

## ONGOING RANDOMIZED CLINICAL TRIALS: THE FUTURE

A search of ClinicalTrials.gov and other public reporting databases (as of September 28,

2018) indicates that there are 4 ongoing randomized clinical trials will provide further inside into the benefits of CA in patients with HFrEF.

The first of these 4 trials is the Atrial Fibrillation Management in Congestive Heart Failure With Ablation trial (AMICA; NCT00652522). AMICA will compare ablation with medical therapy, including rate and rhythm control in 202 patients with persistent AF, LVEF less than 35%, and ICD or CRT-D. The primary endpoint is, again, improvement in LV function as measured by LVEF on echocardiography at 1 year. A second trial, the Atrial Fibrillation Ablation Compared to Rate Control Strategy in Patients With Impaired Left Ventricular Function trial (AFARC-LVF; NCT02509754) will enroll 180 subjects with LVEF less than 35% and persistent AF and randomize them to CA or a rate control strategy. The primary endpoint in AFARC-LVF will be a composite of the improvement of LVEF greater than 35% and NYHA class lower than II at 6 months. Although the results of these 2 trials are highly anticipated, they are again limited by the use of surrogate endpoints, specifically, improvement in LV function and symptoms that may help support or contradict the results of the previous "proof-of-concept" clinical trials through their bigger sample sizes.

There are also ongoing randomized trials that will focus on cardiovascular outcomes. Similar to the previously published AATAC trial, the ongoing CATCH AF (Catheter Ablation vs Medical Therapy in Congested Hearts With AF; NCT02686749) trial will compare CA with AAD therapy. CATCH AF will enroll 220 patients with symptomatic AF and LVEF 24% to 45%. The primary endpoint is a composite of first hospitalization for HF, recurrence of AF, or direct current cardioversion, but with a follow-up of only 1 year.

Rhythm Control-Catheter Ablation With or Without Anti-arrhythmic Drug Control of Maintaining Sinus Rhythm vs Rate Control With Medical Therapy and/or Atrio-ventricular Junction Ablation and Pacemaker Treatment for Atrial Fibrillation trial (RAFT AF; NCT01420393) is the largest ongoing trial with a "hard" endpoint composite of all-cause mortality and HF hospitalization. The trial has randomized 412 patients to receive ablation or rate control, which is much less than the 1000 and then 600 patients initially targeted. Patients enrolled had AF and symptomatic HF, stratified for preserved (LVEF >45%) or impaired (LVEF <45%). Because of the stratification by EF, the trial may be the first to offer insights into the role of ablation in patients with AF and HFpEF.

## UNMET NEEDS FOR ATRIAL FIBRILLATION ABLATION IN HEART FAILURE PATIENTS: WHAT CAN WE DO?

To date, randomized clinical trials have proven the concept that ablation may be effective for treatment of AF in patients with HFrEF, showing improvement in QoL, symptoms, and LVEF, as well as better maintenance of sinus rhythm. However, only one trial (CASTLE-AF) was designed with adequate power and prolonged follow-up in order to assess harder outcomes, including hospitalization and survival. Like most randomized trials, the enrolled population was highly selected. Therefore, at most, it might be concluded that in carefully selected patients who remain symptomatic with HFrEF and AF despite optimal medical therapy, who have already failed AAD attempts to maintain sinus rhythm, and who have been optimized with device therapy (ICD and/or CRT), ablation may offer a benefit in reduction of hospitalization and/or mortality. Of course, outside of patients who have these characteristics, there are many patients with AF and HF in whom it is unknown if CA improves outcomes.[22]

The first unaddressed question is whether these results of ablation will be durable. It is well appreciated that HF is a progressive disease, and as it progresses, the pathologic changes in the atria also worsen, increasing the risk of recurrent AF. Among the completed clinical trials, the longest follow-up was 37.8 months (CASTLE-AF); however, most of the trials had follow-up ≤2 years, and most of them were limited to 6 months. All of the trials also demonstrated that more than one procedure was required in many patients to maintain sinus rhythm. If follow-up were continued, would even more ablations be required? Is there a point of no return, where further ablation will offer no further benefit? This question is critical, because if ablation cannot offer a durable effect, then can one count on the approach being cost-effective?

The second unaddressed question is that of patient selection. Who is the optimal patient for receiving AF ablation in the setting of HF? To date, all of the trials have focused on patients with HFrEF. However, there are even greater numbers of elderly patients with HFpEF, and there is almost no clinical trial evidence demonstrating the impact of ablation for these patients. Limited observational data suggest that the benefits may be similar in patients with AF and HFpEF.[23] Although CABANA and CAFT AF may offer some preliminary insights, neither study was designed or powered to determine the efficacy of ablation in these patients. Because these patients with HFpEF are often quite elderly with multiple comorbidities, it is unclear if ablation would be optimal in these patients. Future randomized trials focused exclusively on HFpEF are going to be critical if ablation will ever be used broadly in the treatment of HF.

Although there are supportive data in patients with HFrEF, who are the best candidates? As the EF continues to decline, the benefits of ablation may be eclipsed by other risks. What is the appropriate cutoff for EF, left atrial size, and other parameters of frailty before the thought of ablation is abandoned? Do patients need to fail AAD treatment first, or can ablation be offered as first-line therapy for selected patients. Again, only larger randomized trials with adequate numbers of high-risk patients will ever answer these questions. Then, there is the broader question of how to identify HF patients in whom AF is definitely a contributing factor versus those in whom AF may just be a "bystander." Perhaps a trial of sinus rhythm (whether by cardioversion and/or antiarrhythmics) can truly identify those in whom elimination of AF may benefit, and these carefully selected patients may need to be the target population for future clinical trials.

The third major unaddressed question is that of the optimal ablation strategy in patients with AF and HF. Most of these patients have persistent or long-standing persistent AF. Even if they have paroxysmal AF, the atrial and ventricular substrate may be sufficiently advanced that PVI alone may not be sufficient. Nevertheless, PVI is the only strategy that has been proven to be of benefit for AF ablation. Additional ablation, such as empiric linear ablation or ablation of continuous fractionated electrograms, may offer no additional benefit beyond PVI alone, as demonstrated by the STAR AF II trial.[24] Newer approaches for ablation of persistent AF, such as targeting rotational activations, low-voltage regions, or non-PV triggers remain untested in larger randomized trials. If the method of ablation cannot be agreed upon, then how can one expect to optimize outcomes of ablation in patients with advanced substrates?

The technique of ablation also relates directly to the potential complications. Overall, recent registries and clinical trials have demonstrated a decline in procedural complications.[10,25] However, these results are largely in younger, healthier patients, and the potential risks in populations with significant comorbidities such as HF patients are not really known. Trials to date have shown a large range in complications from 2.9% in the ATAAC trial to 27% in MacDonald and colleagues. Even in the most recent CASTLE-AF, procedural complications were reported in 8.4% of the patients, including a 1.7% rate of cardiac tamponade and 1.7% rate of major bleeding, which is significantly higher than the rates reported in recent registries that included healthier patients with preserved LVEF.[10,25]

Perhaps newer ablation technologies can improve safety sufficiently to address the HF population, whether it be radiofrequency optimized with contact force measurements, "one-shot" balloon-based technologies (such as cryothermy or laser), or novel technologies like electroporation. Also, one cannot forget that the long-term side effects of AADs are significant too. In patients with HF, guideline-recommended AAD therapy is limited to dofetilide and amiodarone. Sotalol can be used with precaution, but it is contraindicated in patients with kidney insufficiency, which usually coexists with HF.[12] Amiodarone is the most common AAD used in these patients, but it is associated with a higher risk of toxicity, including thyroid, skin, lung, neurologic, and eye, and also bradycardia in HF patients,[26] which was up to 44.5% in the DIONYSOS trial.[11]

With all of the unknowns, it is clear that many more trials are needed to answer the question of whether maintenance of sinus rhythm with ablation can benefit patients with HFrEF, HFpEF, and AF. In the meantime, what can be recommended? The authors think that CA should be used selectively in patients with HF and AF. First, patients should already be optimized with HF medical therapy, oral anticoagulation, AF rate control, and if necessary, ICD and/or CRT therapy before ablation is considered. Second, patients must be carefully selected to avoid patients with high frailty in whom ablation may cause more procedural harm than long-term good. Third, a trial of sinus rhythm by cardioversion and/or drugs should be attempted. Even if the time in sinus rhythm is brief, it may be long enough to determine if there is improvement in the patient's symptoms and functional status. Patients who are recurrently hospitalized because of episodes of AF and in whom AF is thought to be the primary cause of cardiomyopathy ("rate-related") may be particularly suited for ablation. Finally, patients, operators, and referring physicians must understand that more than one procedure may be required in order to maintain sinus rhythm (with or without ongoing AAD therapy) and that the benefit may not be realized for months (**Fig. 1**).

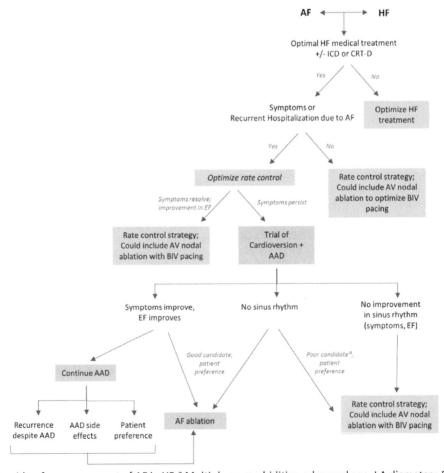

**Fig. 1.** Algorithm for management of AF in HF. [a] Multiple co-morbidities, advanced age, LA diameter >55–60 mm, very low EF. AV, atrioventricular; BIV, biventricular.

## SUMMARY

Randomized clinical trials have reported a significant improvement in symptoms, QoL, and EF in patients with HFrEF who underwent a CA for paroxysmal or persistent AF. However, further studies with hard endpoints like mortality and hospitalization are warranted to be able to generalize the invasive approach to most of these patients, especially considering the lower success rate and higher incidence of adverse events reported compared with a healthier population.

## REFERENCES

1. Kotecha D, Holmes J, Krum H, et al. Efficacy of β blockers in patients with heart failure plus atrial fibrillation: an individual-patient data meta-analysis. Lancet 2014;384:2235–43.

2. Mamas MA, Caldwell JC, Chacko S, et al. A meta-analysis of the prognostic significance of atrial fibrillation in chronic heart failure. Eur J Heart Fail 2009; 11:676–83.

3. Wang TJ, Larson MG, Levy D, et al. Temporal relations of atrial fibrillation and congestive heart failure and their joint influence on mortality: the Framingham heart study. Circulation 2003;107:2920–5.

4. Roy D, Talajic M, Dorian P, et al. Amiodarone to prevent recurrence of atrial fibrillation. Canadian trial of atrial fibrillation Investigators. N Engl J Med 2010; 342:913–20.

5. Torp-Pedersen C, Møller M, Bloch-Thomsen, et al. Dofetilide in patients with congestive heart failure and left ventricular dysfunction. Danish Investigations of Arrhythmia and Mortality on Dofetilide Study Group. N Engl J Med 1999;341:857–65.

6. Wazni OM, Marrouche NF, Martin DO, et al. Radiofrequency ablation vs antiarrhythmic drugs as first-line treatment of symptomatic atrial fibrillation: a randomized trial. J Am Med Assoc 2005;293:2634–40.

7. Cosedis Nielsen J, Johannessen A, Raatikainen P, et al. Radiofrequency ablation as initial therapy in paroxysmal atrial fibrillation. N Engl J Med 2012; 367:1587–95.

8. Morillo CA, Verma A, Connolly SJ, et al. Radiofrequency ablation vs antiarrhythmic drugs as first-line treatment of paroxysmal atrial fibrillation (RAAFT-2) a randomized trial. JAMA 2014;311:692–9.

9. Arbelo E, Brugada J, Blomström-Lundqvist C, et al. Contemporarymanagement of patients undergoing atrial fibrillation ablation: inhospital and 1-year follow-up findings from the ESC-EHRA atrial fibrillation ablation long-term registry. Eur Heart J 2017;38:1303–16.

10. Mansour M, Lakkireddy D, Packer D, et al. Safety of catheter ablation of atrial fibrillation using fiber optic–based contact force sensing. Hear Rhythm 2017;14:1631–6.

11. Le Heuzey JY, De Ferrari GM, Radzik D, et al. A short-term, randomized, double-blind, parallel-group study to evaluate the efficacy and safety of dronedarone versus amiodarone in patients with persistent atrial fibrillation: the dionysos study. J Cardiovasc Electrophysiol 2010;21:597–605.

12. January CT, Wann LS, Alpert JS, et al. 2014 AHA/ACC/HRS guideline for the management of patients with atrial fibrillation: executive summary: a report of the American college of cardiology/American heart association task force on practice guidelines and the heart rhythm society. J Am Coll Cardiol 2014; 64:2245–80.

13. Anselmino M, Matta M, D'Ascenzo F, et al. Catheter ablation of atrial fibrillation in patients with left ventricular systolic dysfunction: a systematic review and meta-analysis. Circ Arrhythm Electrophysiol 2014;7:1011–8.

14. Ganesan AN, Nandal S, Lüker J, et al. Catheter ablation of atrial fibrillation in patients with concomitant left ventricular impairment: a systematic review of efficacy and effect on ejection fraction. Hear Lung Circ 2015;24:270–80.

15. Khan MN, Jaïs P, Cummings J, et al. Pulmonary-vein isolation for atrial fibrillation in patients with heart failure. N Engl J Med 2008;359:1778–85.

16. Jones DG, Haldar SK, Hussain W, et al. A randomized trial to assess catheter ablation versus rate control in the management of persistent atrial fibrillation in heart failure. J Am Coll Cardiol 2013;61:1894–903.

17. Hunter RJ, Berriman TJ, Diab I, et al. A randomized controlled trial of catheter ablation versus medical treatment of atrial fibrillation in heart failure (the CAMTAF trial). Circ Arrhythmia Electrophysiol 2014; 7:31–8.

18. Prabhu S, Taylor AJ, Costello BT, et al. Catheter ablation versus medical rate control in atrial fibrillation and systolic dysfunction: the CAMERA-MRI Study. J Am Coll Cardiol 2017;70:1949–61.

19. MacDonald MR, Connelly DT, Hawkins NM, et al. Radiofrequency ablation for persistent atrial fibrillation in patients with advanced heart failure and severe left ventricular systolic dysfunction: a randomised controlled trial. Heart 2011;97:740–7.

20. Di Biase L, Mohanty P, Mohanty S, et al. Ablation versus amiodarone for treatment of persistent atrial fibrillation in patients with congestive heart failure and an implanted device: results from the AATAC multicenter randomized trial. Circulation 2016;133: 1637–44.

21. Marrouche NF, Brachmann J, Andresen D, et al. Catheter ablation for atrial fibrillation with heart failure. N Engl J Med 2018;378:417–27.

22. Mathew JS, Marzec LN, Kennedy KF, et al. Atrial fibrillation in heart failure us ambulatory cardiology practices and the potential for uptake of catheter

ablation: an National Cardiovascular Data Registry (NCDR®) Research to Practice (R2P) project. J Am Heart Assoc 2017;6:1–11.

23. Black-Maier E, Ren X, Steinberg BA, et al. Catheter ablation of atrial fibrillation in patients with heart failure and preserved ejection fraction. Hear Rhythm 2018;15:651–7.

24. Verma A, Jiang CY, Betts TR, et al. Approaches to catheter ablation for persistent atrial fibrillation. N Engl J Med 2015;372:1812–22.

25. De Potter T, Van Herendael H, Balasubramaniam R, et al. Safety and long-term effectiveness of paroxysmal atrial fibrillation ablation with a contact force-sensing catheter: real-world experience from a prospective, multicentre observational cohort registry. Europace 2018. https://doi.org/10.1093/europace/eux290.

26. Vorperian VR, Havighurst TC, Miller S, et al. Adverse effects of low dose amiodarone: a meta-analysis. J Am Coll Cardiol 1997;30:791–801.

# Mechanisms of Improved Mortality Following Ablation
## Does Ablation Restore Beta-Blocker Benefit in Atrial Fibrillation/Heart Failure?

T. Jared Bunch, MD[a,b,c],*, Heidi T. May, PhD[a],
Kia Afshar, MD[a,d], Rami Alharethi, MD[a,d], John D. Day, MD[a]

**KEYWORDS**

• Catheter ablation • Atrial fibrillation • Congestive heart failure • Beta-blockers • Mortality

**KEY POINTS**

• Multiple observational trials have shown that atrial fibrillation ablation favorably impacts long-term outcomes in patients with systolic heart failure that have been confirmed by multiple randomized prospective trials.
• Ablation favorably impacts left ventricular function and remodeling, risk of heart failure hospitalization, and to a variable degree mortality.
• Beta-blockers are a cornerstone therapy in patients with chronic systolic heart failure with a reduced ejection fraction, supported by randomized trials.
• Observational data suggest a potential long-term benefit of beta-blockers with ablation that becomes augmented as follow-up is extended.

Beta-adrenergic blockade (beta-blocker) therapy is a cornerstone of treatment in patients with chronic systolic heart failure with a reduced ejection fraction, supported by randomized trials, and endorsed as a Class 1A recommendation in guideline statements.[1,2] Beta-blockers can decrease morbidity and mortality in patients with heart failure and structural heart disease while improving symptoms and quality of life.[3–5] For the purpose of this review, heart failure refers to patients with systolic heart failure with a reduced ejection fraction.

## MECHANISMS OF BETA-BLOCKER BENEFIT IN HEART FAILURE

In patients with heart failure, the sympathetic nervous system is activated and circulating catecholamines are increased. This response occurs early and the severity of catecholamine elevation strongly associates with mortality risk.[6] Catecholamine stimulation impacts the heart through multiple pathways including augmenting heart rate, increasing energy consumption, stimulation of the renin–angiotensin–aldosterone axis, which

Disclosure Statement: Dr T.J. Bunch - research grants from Boehringer Ingelheim and Boston scientific. Dr J.D. Day - consultant and honorarium from Boston Scientific, Abbott Medical.
[a] Intermountain Medical Center Heart Institute, Intermountain Medical Center, 5169 Cottonwood St, Murray, UT 84017, USA; [b] Intermountain Heart Rhythm Specialists, Eccles Outpatient Care Center, Suite 510, Intermountain Medical Center, 5169 Cottonwood St, Murray, UT 84017, USA; [c] Department of Internal Medicine, Stanford University, 300 Pasteur Drive, Palo Alto, CA 94305, USA; [d] Department of Internal Medicine, University of Utah, 30 N 1900 E, Salt Lake City, UT 84132, USA
* Corresponding author. Intermountain Medical Center, Eccles Outpatient Care Center, 5169 Cottonwood Street, Suite 510, Murray, UT 84107.
E-mail address: Thomas.bunch@imail.org

Cardiol Clin 37 (2019) 177–183
https://doi.org/10.1016/j.ccl.2019.01.011
0733-8651/19/© 2019 Elsevier Inc. All rights reserved.

cardiology.theclinics.com

results in adverse remodeling, myocyte hypertrophy, and interstitial fibrosis.[7]

The Beta-Blockers in Heart Failure Collaborative Group has provided evidence of benefit beyond heart rate reduction from pooled individual patient data derived from randomized clinical trials of beta-blockers versus placebo. From this dataset, beta-blockers reduced the average ventricular rate by 12 beats/min. Mortality was significantly reduced (hazard ratio [HR], 0.73; 95% confidence interval [CI], 0.67–0.79). Although a lower heart rate was predictive of lower mortality, the benefit of beta-blockers was observed across multiple heart rate ranges.[8] Treatment with beta-blockers favorably impacts structural function and ventricular remodeling over time. In studies with serial imaging after initiation of beta-blockade with metoprolol or carvedilol, decreases in end-systolic and end-diastolic volumes were found with an average improvement in ejection fraction of approximately of 4% to 5%.[9,10] Additional benefits with beta-blockade are related to restoration of beta-receptor responsiveness. Beta-blockade treatment augments contractile function by enhancing chronotropic and inotropic responsiveness.[11]

## BETA-BLOCKERS AND ARRHYTHMIA IN HEART FAILURE

In addition to structural and hemodynamic benefits, beta-blockers favorably impact arrhythmia risk in patients with heart failure. Beta-blocker use in heart failure results in a significant decrease in sudden cardiac death observed in the MERIT-HF trial (3.9 vs 6.6%)[5] and the CIBIS-II trial (3.6 vs 6.3%).[3] The benefit in ventricular arrhythmia reduction with beta-blocker extends to patients with an implantable cardioverter defibrillators. In pooled data from the Multicenter Automatic Defibrillator Implantation Trial II (MADIT II) and the Sudden Cardiac Death in Heart Failure Trial (SCD-HeFT), the absence of a beta-blocker was significantly associated with a higher risk of appropriate implantable cardioverter-defibrillator shocks (odds ratio [OR], 1.61; 95% CI, 1.23–2.12).[12]

Patients with chronic heart failure are at a significantly increased risk of developing atrial fibrillation (AF). The Framingham Study revealed a 4.5 to 6.0 times increased risk of AF in men and women with heart failure.[13] Both a prior history of AF and new-onset AF have been shown to predict the risk of hospitalization for heart failure, implantable cardioverter-defibrillator therapies, and mortality in patients with heart failure.[14] In a metaanalysis of 7 trials, beta-blocker therapy decreases the risk of new-onset AF from 39 to 28 per 1000 patients/y (relative risk reduction of 27%).[15]

## BETA-BLOCKERS AND CARDIAC FIBROSIS

Central to arrhythmia risk and adverse remodeling is cardiac fibrosis. As described elsewhere in this article, long-term beta-blocker therapy improves cardiac remodeling manifested by the echocardiographic parameters of ejection fraction and end-systolic and end-diastolic dimensions. In addition, long-term beta-blocker therapy decrease the risk of both ventricular and atrial arrhythmias. It seems logical that beta-blockers may favorably impact these outcomes by lowering the risk of cardiac fibrosis in the atrium and ventricle.

Very few studies have examined the impact of beta-blockers on cardiac fibrosis and the fibrotic pathway. In a murine model, exposure to metoprolol slightly increased fibrosis and fibrosis signaling.[16] The authors concluded that the slight increased risk of fibrosis may be offset by the other benefits from catecholamine blockade of metoprolol in heart failure. In a second hypertensive murine model of diastolic heart failure, metoprolol exposure prevented the development of fibrosis and heart failure.[17] These divergent animal studies may provide some insight into the preferential benefit of beta-blocker therapy when use early, rather than late, in heart failure.[18]

## IMPACT OF ATRIAL FIBRILLATION ON BETA-BLOCKER THERAPY FOR HEART FAILURE

The Beta-Blockers in Heart Failure Collaborative Group pooled data highlighted the critical correlation between heart rate and outcomes in patients with heart failure and the value across all heart rate strata of beta-blocker therapy. However, when a comparison was made between those patients in AF and sinus rhythm, 3 significant findings were noted. First, the mortality rates were higher in patients with AF (21% vs 16%) regardless of whether they received beta-blockers or placebo. Second, in patients with AF, beta-blocker therapy did not lower risk of mortality in any heart rate group compared with placebo (HR, 0.97; 95% CI, 0.83–1.14; P = .73). Finally, an increased risk of mortality with higher heart rates was not observed in the AF group in both the initial study and a subsequent analysis that looked at baseline and interim heart rates.[8,19]

In aggregate, 5 large studies have examined this topic (**Fig. 1**). Two metaanalyses from Rienstra and colleagues[20] and Kotecha and colleagues[19] failed to show a mortality benefit with beta-blocker

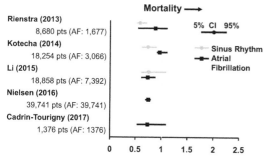

Riemstra (2013)
8,680 pts (AF: 1,677)

Kotecha (2014)
18,254 pts (AF: 3,066)

Li (2015)
18,858 pts (AF: 7,392)

Nielsen (2016)
39,741 pts (AF: 39,741)

Cadrin-Tourigny (2017)
1,376 pts (AF: 1376)

Mortality →

5% CI 95%

Sinus Rhythm
Atrial
Fibrillation

0    0.5    1    1.5    2    2.5

**Fig. 1.** Comparative trials of beta-blocker therapy and atrial fibrillation and mortality risk in patients with heart failure.

therapy in patients with AF. A subanalysis of the AF-CHF trial[21] and 2 national registries[22,23] have shown a mortality benefit with beta-blocker therapy in patients with AF. Multiple knowledge gaps have been identified that may explain the divergent results of these multiple studies. Knowledge gaps exist regarding the optimal dose of beta-blocker therapy, the target heart rate to achieve to observe a potential benefit, whether there is a variance of effect of different beta-blockers, and a potential differential impact of beta-blocker therapy across various stages and severities of heart failure and its comorbidities.

## ANTIARRHYTHMIC DRUG THERAPIES TO IMPROVE BETA-BLOCKER EFFICACY IN HEART FAILURE

In the AF-CHF trial, 1376 patients with an ejection fraction of less than 35% were randomized to rhythm control or rate control; 1085 of the patients (79%) were on a beta-blocker at enrollment. In the rhythm control group, 27% died compared with 25% in the rate control group (*P* = .59).[24] After 12 months in this trial, 82% of patients were on amiodarone therapy and beta-blocker use was significantly lower in patients receiving antiarrhythmic drug therapy (80% vs 88%; *P*<.001). In a propensity-based analysis to account for baseline differences associated with beta-blocker therapy use, beta-blockers were associated with lower all-cause mortality (HR, 0.721; 95% CI, 0.549–0.945; *P* = .0180). There were no significant interactions between beta-blockers and AF subtype or burden. In another subanalysis of the AF-CHF trial that specifically looked at achieved rhythm, in those patients who maintained sinus rhythm, beta-blocker use was associated with a lower risk of mortality (HR, 0.70; 95% CI, 0.55–0.90; *P* = .006).[25]

In the DIAMOND-CHF trial, 1518 patients were randomly assigned to dofetilide or placebo.[26] Over a median follow-up of 18 months, AF-free survival free rates in the dofetilide group were approximately 65% versus 30% in the placebo arm, and there was no difference in mortality. In comparison with the AF-CHF trial, only 12% of patients received beta-blockers. Although treatment with dofetilide was associated with a lower risk of heart failure hospitalization, mortality rates were similar to treatment with placebo (41% vs 42%, respectively).

## CATHETER ABLATION OF ATRIAL FIBRILLATION IN PATIENTS WITH HEART FAILURE

A metaanalysis of 26 studies was performed that included 1838 patients with heart failure and AF that looked to compare outcomes based on treatment with catheter ablation versus medical therapy.[27] The mean age was 59 (range, 51–61) years with a mean ejection fraction of 40% (range, 35%–46%). Beta-blocker use was variable with a mean use of 70% (range, 43%–82%). Over a mean follow-up of 23 months, freedom from arrhythmia recurrences at the end of follow-up period was 60% (range, 54%–67%). Single procedure efficacy ranged from 36% to 44%. The ejection fraction improved significantly during follow-up by 13%, from 40% to 53%.

There are 6 randomized trials that have examined the role of catheter ablation for AF in patients with heart failure versus medical therapy alone.[28–33] In all these trials, mortality rates were similar during short-term follow-up or significantly decreased with extended follow-up in the catheter ablation groups despite AF freedom rates similar to those observed in the metaanalysis. In those trials that specifically looked for heart failure/cardiac hospitalizations, a decrease with catheter ablation was observed versus medical therapy.

Although patients with heart failure who are in sinus rhythm have a lower long-term risks of mortality and heart failure compared with those in AF, antiarrhythmic drugs used as a means to augment the likelihood of sinus rhythm do not improve outcomes. There are multiple potential possibilities to explain the lack of benefit with medical therapies, including toxicities associated with long-term antiarrhythmic drug therapies, poor patient tolerance and compliance, and a lack of efficacy of the available antiarrhythmic drugs. Catheter ablation, when successful, circumvents many of these limitations with antiarrhythmic drugs and, in comparison, results in higher rates of long-term arrhythmia-free

**Table 1**
Randomized clinical trials comparing catheter ablation to medical therapy in patients with heart failure

| Trial | N (Ablation) | Inclusion Criteria | Demographics (Ablation vs Meds) | Follow-up | Primary Endpoint | Freedom From AF | Outcomes (Ablation vs Meds) |
|---|---|---|---|---|---|---|---|
| MacDonald[33] | 41 (22) | Persistent AF, NYHA II-III, EF ≤35% | Age: 62 y vs 64 y EF: 16% vs 20% Beta-blockers: 82% vs 95% ACE/ARB: 95% vs 95% | 6 mo | Change in EF from baseline at 6 mo on cardiac magnetic resonance imaging | 50% (27% repeat procedures) | Deaths: 0% vs 0% EF: +8.26 ± 12.0% vs +1.46 ± 5.9% Three patients with worsening heart failure (total population) |
| CAMTAF Trial (2014)[28] | 50 (26) | NYHA II-IV, EF <50% | Age: 55 ± 12 y vs 60 ± 10 y EF: 32 ± 8 vs 34 ± 12 Beta-blockers: 100% vs 100% ACE/ARB: 100% vs 100% | 12 mo | EF at 6 mo | 73% (mean: 1.7 ± 0.7 procedures) | Deaths: 0% vs 4% EF: 40% ± 12% vs 31% ± 13% |
| ARC-HF (2015)[32] | 52 (26) | NYHA II-III, EF ≤35% | Age: 62 ± 9 y vs 64 ± 10 y EF: 25 ± 7 vs 22 ± 8 Beta-blockers: 92% vs 92% ACE/ARB: 100% vs 96% | 12 mo | Peak $V_{O_2}$ | 69% (19% required additional procedures) | Deaths: 0% vs 0% $V_{O_2}$ increase 2.13 (−0.10 to 4.36 mL/kg/min) vs decrease −0.94 (−2.21 to 0.32 mL/kg/min) |
| AATAC Trial (2016)[29] | 203 (102) | NYHA II-III, EF ≤40% | Age: 62 ± 10 y vs 60 ± 11 y EF: 29 ± 5 vs 30 ± 8 Beta-blockers: 76% vs 80% ACE/ARB: 92% vs 88% | 24 mo | Freedom from AF | 70% (average: 1.4 ± 0.6 procedures) | Deaths: 8% vs 18% Hospitalizations: 31% vs 51% |
| CAMERA-MRI Study (2018)[30] | 68 (33) | Persistent AF, idiopathic cardiomyopathy, EF <45% | Age: 59 ± 11 y vs 62 ± 9.4 y EF: 32 ± 9, 34 ± 8 Beta-blockers: 88% vs 85% ACE/ARB: 94% vs 94% | 6 mo | Change in EF from baseline at 6 mo on cardiac MRI | 56% (single procedure) | Deaths: 0% vs 0% EF: 50 ± 11 vs 39 ± 9 Hospitalizations: 0% vs 12% |
| CASTLE-AF (2018)[31] | 363 (179) | NYHA II-IV heart EF ≤35%, ICD or CRT-D | Age: 64 y vs 64 y EF: 33 vs 33 ACE inhibitor: 94% vs 91% Beta-blockers: 92% vs 95% | ≤60 mo | Composite of death from any cause or worsening of heart failure that led to an unplanned hospitalization | 63% (repeat procedures in 24.5% of patients) | Deaths: 13% vs 25% Composite: 29% vs 45% EF improvement: 8% vs 0.2% |

*Abbreviations:* ACE, angiotensin-converting-enzyme inhibitor; AF, atrial fibrillation; ARB, angiotensin receptor blocker; CRT-D, cardiac resynchronization therapy defibrillator; EF, ejection fraction; ICD, implantable cardioverter-defibrillator; NYHA, New York Heart Association.

survival and lower AF burden rates. For example, as a first-line therapy, catheter ablation compared with medical therapies lowers risk of AF recurrence by 37%.[34]

## DOES CATHETER ABLATION RESTORE BETA-BLOCKER BENEFIT IN PATIENTS WITH HEART FAILURE?

There are several possible mechanisms that suggest that catheter ablation may restore beta-blocker benefit in patients with heart failure. First, because beta-blocker therapy preferentially benefits patients with heart failure in sinus rhythm compared with those in AF, successful ablation should have a role in restoring beta-blocker effectiveness through the maintenance of sinus rhythm. Second, as observed in the AF-CHF trial, beta-blocker use is lower (80% vs 88%) with long-term antiarrhythmic drug exposure when patients are compared with those treated in a rate control strategy alone. Antiarrhythmic drug therapy coupled with beta-blockers can increase side effects such as bradycardia, fatigue, brady-dependent proarrhythmia, and negative inotropy. Also, the complexity of the drug dosing and scheduling decreases compliance rates and increases the potential for drug–drug interactions.

As noted in **Table 1**, in randomized prospective trials of catheter ablation versus medical therapy in patients with heart failure, the use of beta-blockers was very high (76%–100%) with no significant differences in the groups compared. These trial characteristics minimize potential insight into a restorative value of catheter ablation for beta-blocker therapy in patients with heart failure. We are unaware of observational data comparing catheter ablation in patients with heart failure treated with and without beta-blocker therapy.

To the look at a potentially favorable impact of catheter ablation on beta-blocker therapy impact, we explored arrhythmia and heart failure long-term outcomes in the Intermountain Medical Center database in patients with AF and chronic systolic heart failure with an ejection fraction of less than 35%. The patients with and without ablation were matched 1:3 by age (within 2 years), sex, and $CHA_2DS_2$-Vasc score. Patients were further stratified by receiving or not receiving a beta-blocker. Four groups were compared: AF ablation patients without a beta-blocker (n = 56), AF ablation patients with a beta-blocker (n = 195), no AF ablation patients without a beta-blocker (n = 297), and no AF ablation patients with a beta-blocker (n = 728). The average age of the AF ablation group was 66 ± 12 years versus 68.5 ± 13 years in the AF nonablation group (P = .02) and 78% were male in each group. The ejection fraction was 27.4 ± 5.9 in the ablation versus 26.6 ± 6.6 in the no ablation group (P = .08). The 1- and 5-year outcomes are displayed in **Figs. 2** and **3**, respectively.

At 1 year in the ablation group, beta-blocker therapy was associated with a 2.1% increase in death and, in the no AF ablation group, a 21.3% decrease in death. Hospitalization for heart failure was decreased by 4.9% in the AF ablation group and by 2.0% in the non–AF ablation group with beta-blocker therapy. AF recurrence rates were similar at 1 year. When outcomes are extended to 5 years total mortality, cardiovascular mortality, and heart failure hospitalization were all decreased in the beta-blocker AF ablation group with the magnitude of benefit greater than in the nonablation group. These beneficial hard end points were observed despite higher recurrence rates of AF in both the ablation and nonablation groups in patients who had received beta-blockers. These observational data provide early

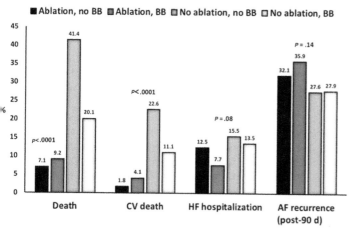

Fig. 2. One-year outcomes of atrial fibrillation patients compared by ablation and beta-blocker use.

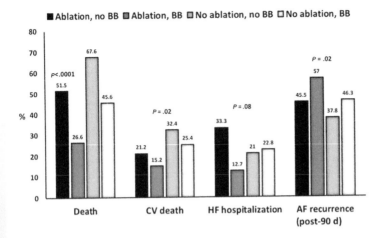

**Ablation, no BB** **Ablation, BB** **No ablation, no BB** **No ablation, BB**

**Fig. 3.** Five-year outcomes of atrial fibrillation patients compared by ablation and beta-blocker use.

evidence of a potential synergistic benefit of beta-blocker therapy and ablation, particularly manifesting as these patients with heart failure are followed long-term.

## SUMMARY

Multiple observational trials have shown that AF ablation favorably impacts long-term outcomes in patients with systolic heart failure. These observational trial outcomes have been confirmed by multiple randomized prospective trials that have highlighted the favorably impact of ablation on left ventricular function and remodeling, risk of heart failure hospitalization, and to a variable degree mortality. The mechanisms behind the observed benefits are likely multifactorial because AF recurrences after ablation remain high and multiple ablation procedures are often required.

The concept of ablation as a synergistic strategy with established heart failure medications is new and supported conceptually by the value of restoring sinus rhythm, avoidance of long-term antiarrhythmic drug therapies, and minimization of drug–drug interactions that may influence the use or titration of guideline supported therapies for heart failure. Our institutional experience data suggest a potential long-term benefit of beta-blockers with ablation that becomes augmented as follow-up is extended from 1 to 5 years.

## REFERENCES

1. McMurray JJ, Adamopoulos S, Anker SD, et al, ESC Committee for Practice Guidelines. ESC guidelines for the diagnosis and treatment of acute and chronic heart failure 2012: the task force for the diagnosis and treatment of acute and chronic heart failure 2012 of the European Society of Cardiology. Developed in collaboration with the Heart Failure Association (HFA) of the ESC. Eur Heart J 2012;33: 1787–847.
2. Yancy CW, Jessup M, Bozkurt B, et al, American College of Cardiology Foundation, American Heart Association Task Force on Practice Guidelines. 2013 ACCF/AHA guideline for the management of heart failure: a report of the American College of Cardiology Foundation/American Heart Association Task Force on practice guidelines. J Am Coll Cardiol 2013;62:e147–239.
3. The cardiac insufficiency bisoprolol study II (CIBIS-II): a randomised trial. Lancet 1999;353:9–13.
4. Packer M, Bristow MR, Cohn JN, et al. The effect of carvedilol on morbidity and mortality in patients with chronic heart failure. U.S. Carvedilol Heart Failure Study Group. N Engl J Med 1996;334:1349–55.
5. Effect of metoprolol CR/XL in chronic heart failure: metoprolol CR/XL randomised intervention trial in congestive heart failure (MERIT-HF). Lancet 1999; 353:2001–7.
6. Cohn JN, Levine TB, Olivari MT, et al. Plasma norepinephrine as a guide to prognosis in patients with chronic congestive heart failure. N Engl J Med 1984;311:819–23.
7. Sackner-Bernstein JD, Mancini DM. Rationale for treatment of patients with chronic heart failure with adrenergic blockade. JAMA 1995;274:1462–7.
8. Kotecha D, Flather MD, Altman DG, et al, Beta Blockers in Heart Failure Collaborative Group. Heart rate and rhythm and the benefit of beta-blockers in patients with heart failure. J Am Coll Cardiol 2017; 69:2885–96.
9. Groenning BA, Nilsson JC, Sondergaard L, et al. Anti remodeling effects on the left ventricle during beta blockade with metoprolol in the treatment of chronic heart failure. J Am Coll Cardiol 2000;36:2072–80.
10. Chatterjee S, Biondi-Zoccai G, Abbate A, et al. Benefits of beta blockers in patients with heart failure and reduced ejection fraction: network meta-analysis. BMJ 2013;346:f55.

11. Gilbert EM, Abraham WT, Olsen S, et al. Comparative hemodynamic, left ventricular functional, and antiadrenergic effects of chronic treatment with metoprolol versus carvedilol in the failing heart. Circulation 1996;94:2817–25.

12. Zeitler EP, Al-Khatib SM, Friedman DJ, et al. Predicting appropriate shocks in patients with heart failure: patient level meta-analysis from SCD-HeFT and MADIT II. J Cardiovasc Electrophysiol 2017;28:1345–51.

13. Kannel WB, Wolf PA, Benjamin EJ, et al. Prevalence, incidence, prognosis, and predisposing conditions for atrial fibrillation: population-based estimates. Am J Cardiol 1998;82:2N–9N.

14. Bunch TJ, Day JD, Olshansky B, et al, INTRINSIC RV Study Investigators. Newly detected atrial fibrillation in patients with an implantable cardioverter-defibrillator is a strong risk marker of increased mortality. Heart Rhythm 2009;6:2–8.

15. Nasr IA, Bouzamondo A, Hulot JS, et al. Prevention of atrial fibrillation onset by beta-blocker treatment in heart failure: a meta-analysis. Eur Heart J 2007;28:457–62.

16. Nakaya M, Chikura S, Watari K, et al. Induction of cardiac fibrosis by beta-blocker in G protein-independent and G protein-coupled receptor kinase 5/beta-arrestin2-dependent Signaling pathways. J Biol Chem 2012;287:35669–77.

17. Kobayashi M, Machida N, Mitsuishi M, et al. Beta-blocker improves survival, left ventricular function, and myocardial remodeling in hypertensive rats with diastolic heart failure. Am J Hypertens 2004;17:1112–9.

18. Bristow MR. beta-adrenergic receptor blockade in chronic heart failure. Circulation 2000;101:558–69.

19. Kotecha D, Holmes J, Krum H, et al, Beta-Blockers in Heart Failure Collaborative Group. Efficacy of beta blockers in patients with heart failure plus atrial fibrillation: an individual-patient data meta-analysis. Lancet 2014;384:2235–43.

20. Rienstra M, Damman K, Mulder BA, et al. Beta-blockers and outcome in heart failure and atrial fibrillation: a meta-analysis. JACC Heart Fail 2013;1:21–8.

21. Cadrin-Tourigny J, Shohoudi A, Roy D, et al. Decreased mortality with beta-blockers in patients with heart failure and coexisting atrial fibrillation: an AF-CHF substudy. JACC Heart Fail 2017;5:99–106.

22. Li SJ, Sartipy U, Lund LH, et al. Prognostic significance of resting heart rate and use of beta-blockers in atrial fibrillation and sinus rhythm in patients with heart failure and reduced ejection fraction: findings from the Swedish Heart Failure registry. Circ Heart Fail 2015;8:871–9.

23. Nielsen PB, Larsen TB, Gorst-Rasmussen A, et al. beta-blockers in atrial fibrillation patients with or without heart failure: association with mortality in a nationwide cohort study. Circ Heart Fail 2016;9:e002597.

24. Roy D, Talajic M, Nattel S, et al, Atrial Fibrillation and Congestive Heart Failure Investigators. Rhythm control versus rate control for atrial fibrillation and heart failure. N Engl J Med 2008;358:2667–77.

25. Talajic M, Khairy P, Levesque S, et al, AF-CHF Investigators. Maintenance of sinus rhythm and survival in patients with heart failure and atrial fibrillation. J Am Coll Cardiol 2010;55:1796–802.

26. Torp-Pedersen C, Moller M, Bloch-Thomsen PE, et al. Dofetilide in patients with congestive heart failure and left ventricular dysfunction. Danish Investigations of Arrhythmia and Mortality on Dofetilide Study Group. N Engl J Med 1999;341:857–65.

27. Anselmino M, Matta M, D'Ascenzo F, et al. Catheter ablation of atrial fibrillation in patients with left ventricular systolic dysfunction: a systematic review and meta-analysis. Circ Arrhythm Electrophysiol 2014;7:1011–8.

28. Hunter RJ, Berriman TJ, Diab I, et al. A randomized controlled trial of catheter ablation versus medical treatment of atrial fibrillation in heart failure (the CAMTAF trial). Circ Arrhythm Electrophysiol 2014;7:31–8.

29. Di Biase L, Mohanty P, Mohanty S, et al. Ablation versus amiodarone for treatment of persistent atrial fibrillation in patients with congestive heart failure and an implanted device: results from the AATAC multicenter randomized trial. Circulation 2016;133:1637–44.

30. Prabhu S, Taylor AJ, Costello BT, et al. Catheter ablation versus medical rate control in atrial fibrillation and systolic dysfunction: the CAMERA-MRI Study. J Am Coll Cardiol 2017;70:1949–61.

31. Marrouche NF, Brachmann J, Andresen D, et al, CASTLE-AF Investigators. Catheter ablation for atrial fibrillation with heart failure. N Engl J Med 2018;378:417–27.

32. Jones DG, Haldar SK, Hussain W, et al. A randomized trial to assess catheter ablation versus rate control in the management of persistent atrial fibrillation in heart failure. J Am Coll Cardiol 2013;61:1894–903.

33. MacDonald MR, Connelly DT, Hawkins NM, et al. Radiofrequency ablation for persistent atrial fibrillation in patients with advanced heart failure and severe left ventricular systolic dysfunction: a randomised controlled trial. Heart 2011;97:740–7.

34. Hakalahti A, Biancari F, Nielsen JC, et al. Radiofrequency ablation vs. antiarrhythmic drug therapy as first line treatment of symptomatic atrial fibrillation: systematic review and meta-analysis. Europace 2015;17:370–8.

# Atrial Fibrillation Ablation Should Be First-line Therapy in Patients with Heart Failure Reduced Ejection Fraction

Pradyumna Agasthi, MD[a], Andrew Tseng, MD[b], Justin Z. Lee, MBBS[a], Siva K. Mulpuru, MD[c],*

## KEYWORDS

- Atrial fibrillation • Catheter ablation • Mortality • Pharmacologic therapy
- Heart failure hospitalization

## KEY POINTS

- Catheter ablation for atrial fibrillation in patients with heart failure with reduced ejection fraction is effective in maintaining sinus rhythm.
- Multiple ablations might be needed to maintain long-term arrhythmia-free survival.
- Newer technologies have improved safety and efficacy of performing ablation procedures.
- Catheter ablation improves his quality of life, left ventricular function, and all-cause mortality in patients with heart failure with reduced ejection fraction.
- The evidence to support the efficacy of catheter ablation in heart failure with preserved ejection fraction is limited.

## INTRODUCTION

Atrial fibrillation (AF) remains one of the major causes of heart failure, stroke, and cardiovascular morbidity, with an estimated prevalence of 40 million worldwide. The incidence of AF is higher in developed countries, and it is estimated that 1 in 4 middle-aged adults in the United States and Europe has AF.[1] The increased prevalence of AF is predominantly attributed to better detection of silent AF, longer life span, and other conditions predisposing to AF.[2–5] Heart failure and AF are among the 2 major epidemics in cardiovascular medicine contributing to the increased morbidity and mortality, especially when they occur simultaneously in this same patient.[5–7] Presence of underlying heart failure increases the risk of incident AF by 4-fold to 5-fold, especially with the progressive decline in functional capacity as assessed by New York Heart Association (NYHA) functional class.[8,9] Heart failure with preserved ejection fraction (HFpEF) is seen in approximately 50% of patients with chronic heart failure and is associated predominantly with hypertension, older age, and female gender. Prevalence of AF is higher in patients with HFpEF compared with patients with heart failure with reduced ejection fraction (HFrEF).[10–12] Restoration and maintenance of sinus rhythm is a therapeutic intervention commonly performed to improve patient outcomes. Multiple

Disclosure Statement: None of the coauthors have any disclosures.
a Department of Cardiovascular Diseases, Mayo Clinic, 5777 East Mayo Boulevard, Phoenix, AZ 85054, USA;
b Department of Internal Medicine, Mayo Clinic, 5777 East Mayo Boulevard, Phoenix, AZ 85054, USA;
c Department of Cardiovascular Diseases, Mayo Clinic, 200 1st Street Southwest, Rochester, MN 55905, USA
* Corresponding author.
E-mail address: Mulpuru.Siva@mayo.edu

randomized controlled trials have shown, however, that antiarrhythmic drugs lack significant benefit because adverse effects of antiarrhythmic drugs counterbalance the benefit of sinus rhythm maintenance, especially in patients with heart failure.[13–19] Therefore, catheter ablation has been proposed as an alternate means of establishing sinus rhythm in a patient with AF and chronic heart failure, thereby avoiding the long-term risks of antiarrhythmic drug therapy.

The purpose of this article is to review the current evidence and literature evaluating the clinical impact, safety, and efficacy of catheter ablation on clinical outcomes in patients with AF and chronic heart failure.

## PATHOPHYSIOLOGY AND INTERPLAY BETWEEN ATRIAL FIBRILLATION AND HEART FAILURE

AF and HFrEF have similar predisposing risk factors, including diabetes mellitus, hypertension, valvular heart disease, ischemic heart disease, and old age. The progression of AF and HFrEF is interdependent, which can be explained by several mechanisms. Diastolic filling time plays a major role in determining cardiac output. Up to 25% reduction in cardiac output is noted in patients with AF due to irregular ventricular response with variable diastolic filling time. The diastolic filling during long cycles does not compensate for the reduced diastolic filling during the short cycle.[20,21] The loss of atrial kick and its contribution to the ventricular filling decreases the overall cardiac output. It was previously hypothesized that atria potentially lose meaningful contractile function before developing AF. In patients with AF, the atria transiently compensate by improving the atrial reservoir and conduit function in an attempt to compensate for the loss of cardiac output. Eventually, these functions deteriorate due to progressive atrial fibrosis.[22] The reduction in cardiac output leads to up-regulation of neurohormonal vasoconstrictor pathway, including increased endothelin and epinephrine levels typically observed in heart failure.[23–25] AF leads to functional mitral regurgitation secondary to progressive mitral annular dilatation, both in patients with and without a prior history of structural heart disease.[26] Tachycardia-mediated cardiomyopathy is frequently seen in patients with AF with inadequate rate control characterized by a systolic and diastolic dysfunction followed by left ventricular (LV) remodeling. The systolic function often improves with appropriate rate control therapy; however, the diastolic dysfunction persists along with LV hypertrophy.[27–29] Proposed mechanisms of tachycardia-mediated cardiomyopathy include impaired coronary flow reserve, abnormal cardiac calcium handling, myocardial images depletion, extracellular matrix, and myocyte remodeling.[28,30]

Conversely, chronic heart failure promotes progression of AF via neuroendocrine, ultrastructural, and microstructural processes. Chronically elevated left atrial pressures in patients with heart failure leads to remodeling and fibrosis of the left atrial architecture, subsequently serving as a substrate for AF.[31] Areas subjected to high atrial stress frequently show left atrial voltage abnormalities in patients with persistent AF.[32] Persistent upregulation of the renin-angiotensin-aldosterone axis also promotes atrial fibrosis.

## PHARMACOLOGIC THERAPY (RATE VS RHYTHM CONTROL)

AF in patients with congestive heart failure predisposes these patients to poor outcomes; therefore, it seems intuitive to expect improvement in clinical outcomes with the restoration of sinus rhythm. Multiple studies have shown, however, the lack of superiority of pharmacologic rhythm control strategies in comparison to rate control strategy on clinical outcomes.

Caldeira and colleagues[33] performed a systematic review evaluating 8 randomized controlled trials, consisting of 7499 patients, comparing the rate control strategy to pharmacologic rhythm control strategy in patients with persistent AF. No significant difference in cardiovascular mortality (relative risk [RR] 0.99; CI, 0.87–1.13), all-cause mortality (RR 0.95; CI, 0.86–1.05), or sudden cardiac death (RR 1.12; CI, 0.91–1.38) was noted. Only 1 trial was performed, however, specifically in patients with chronic heart failure.

The Rhythm Control versus Rate Control for Atrial Fibrillation and Heart Failure trial performed by Roy and colleagues[17] randomized patients with symptomatic heart failure (NYHA classes II–IV) and AF (67% persistent, 33% paroxysmal) to pharmacologic rhythm control (predominantly amiodarone versus pharmacologic rate control. They enrolled 1376 patients in the trial on guideline-directed heart failure therapy with greater than 90% use of β blockers, angiotensinogen-converting enzyme (ACE) inhibitors, and warfarin. No difference in all cause mortality (hazard ratio [HR] 0.97; 95% CI 0.80–1.17; $P = .73$), cardiovascular mortality (HR 1.06; 95% CI, 0.86–1.30; $P = .59$), or worsening heart failure (HR 0.87; 95% CI, 0.72–1.06 $P = .17$) was noted between both groups, which was similar to the AFFIRM (Atrial Fibrillation Follow-up Investigation of Rhythm Management trial.[34] Although the trials have suggested the lack of benefit of pharmacologic rhythm control strategy, it is important to understand the limitations to the generalizability of the results. These trials were conducted to assess the efficacy of rhythm control and relatively asymptomatic patients, and the impact of recruitment bias in the AFFIRM trial, which enrolled only 54% of the screened patients, cannot be understated. The side effects of antiarrhythmic drugs, including cardiac (conduction block, proarrhythmia, and negative inotropy) and noncardiac toxicities affected the results of the trials.

According to 2014 American Heart Association/American College of Cardiology/Heart Rhythm Society guidelines,[35] the choices of antiarrhythmic drugs in AF were limited to amiodarone and dofetilide in patients with HFrEF. Dronedarone increases early mortality in patients with LV ejection fraction (LVEF) less than 40% or NYHA classes III and IV and, therefore, is contraindicated.[36] The negative inotropic effects of class IC agents per Vaughan-Williams classification are detrimental to patients with HFrEF and, therefore, should be avoided.[35] The efficacy of dofetilide was tested in the DIAMOND-CHF (Danish Investigators of Arrhythmia and Mortality on Dofetilide-congestive heart failure) trial, which included 1518 patients with HFrEF. Compared with placebo, dofetilide was more efficacious in converting patients to sinus rhythm and reduced the risk of heart failure hospitalization (RR 0.75; 95% CI, 0.63–0.89); however, no difference in all-cause mortality was noted.[37] In patients with normal baseline QTc, slight mortality benefit was noted in patients treated with dofetilide and a subsequent post hoc analysis.[38] Amiodarone is by far the most widely used antiarrhythmic agent in patients with chronic heart failure and its use is associated with increased risk of neurologic (4.6% vs 1.9%; $P = .026$), skin (2.3% vs 0.7%; $P = .05$), eye (1.5% vs 0.1; $P = .02$), pulmonary (1.9% vs 0.7%; $P = .073$), and thyroid (3.7% vs 0.4%; $P = .001$) toxicities. Therefore, the benefit of sinus rhythm restoration in patients with heart failure and AF are mitigated by the side effects of antiarrhythmic drugs in this population.

β-Blockers are the cornerstone of medical therapies in patients with HFrEF. The coexistence of AF, however, seems to mitigate the beneficial effect of β-blockers in patients with HFrEF.[39] Studies have shown that the survival benefits of β-blockers are seen only in patients who are in sinus rhythm.[40,41] Multiple meta-analyses of randomized clinical trials evaluating the efficacy of β-blockers in comparison to a placebo control in patients with HFrEF and AF have shown significant reduction and

cardiovascular hospitalizations and all-cause mortality in patients in sinus rhythm but not in AF, despite a similar degree of ventricular rate control.[41,42] This was a premise for evaluating the efficacy of catheter ablation to maintain sinus rhythm in this population by avoiding the side effects of antiarrhythmic drug therapy.

## CATHETER ABLATION FOR ATRIAL FIBRILLATION

Maintenance of sinus rhythm in patients with heart failure and AF was previously shown associated with decreased all-cause and heart failure hospitalizations and improved mortality.[43] The optimal strategy for rhythm control, however, remains open to discussion. The treatment strategy should be individualized by balancing the potential risks of intraprocedural complications with the long-term benefit of successful ablation. There is a growing body of literature supporting catheter ablation compared with antiarrhythmic drug therapy for patients with chronic heart failure.[44–46] This led to the updated recommendations in the 2017 Heart Rhythm Society/European Heart Rhythm Association/European Cardiac Arrhythmia Society/Asia Pacific Heart Rhythm Society/Latin American Society of Cardiac Stimulation and Electrophysiology expert consensus statement, giving a class IIa (level of evidence B-R) recommendation to pursue AF ablation in selected patients with heart failure.[47] In contemporary practice, ablation strategy typically targets initiating triggers (ie, pulmonary veins) and left atrial tissue that is electrically active and sustains perpetuation of AF. Therefore, circumferential lesions are placed outside the pulmonary veins within the left atrial myocardium, with a goal of electrical pulmonary vein isolation, which may be adequate in patients with paroxysmal AF. In patients with chronic heart failure or persistent AF, however, the presence of progressive left atrial fibrosis and enlargement results in nonpulmonary vein triggers as well as shift and the AF perpetuation sites beyond the junction of the pulmonary vein and left atrium. Therefore, additional ablation strategies, such as ablation of complex fractionated atrial electrograms or rotors, posterior wall isolation, empirical linear ablation, targeting nonpulmonary vein triggers, and scar-based ablation, have been proposed. Although the incremental benefit of these strategies on top of traditional pulmonary vein isolation remains currently uncertain, novel innovations in the field of electrophysiology and catheter-based therapy will help advance and refine the overall strategy of ablation as well as help tailor approach based on individual patient characteristics.[47–56]

Current guidelines lack recommendations regarding patient selection for catheter ablation in heart failure population. Typically, ideal patients for AF ablation are otherwise healthy individuals with high symptom burden in whom optimal arrhythmia-free survival can be obtained. They are underrepresented, however, in a population with heart failure, especially due to presence underlying structural heart disease like left atrial dilatation, which is associated with recurrent AF after catheter ablation, requiring additional ablation procedures in up to 40% to 50% of the patients to obtain long-term arrhythmia-free survival.[47,57,58] Left atrial size and volume are dynamic and are affected by multiple factors likely volume status, rate control, and rhythm. Therefore, it remains challenging to define a cutoff beyond which ablation should not be performed.[59] In addition to left atrial volume, persistent AF, decreased LVEF, and increased left atrial diameter have shown associated with recurrence of AF after catheter ablation procedures.[47,60]

## IMPACT OF CATHETER ABLATION IN HEART FAILURE WITH REDUCED EJECTION FRACTION

The frequency of catheter ablation for AF in patients with HFrEF has increased despite the uncertainty regarding the optimal ablation technique. Evidence for catheter ablation has progressed from small observational studies to large multicenter randomized controlled trials testing the efficacy of catheter ablation in comparison to pharmacologic (rate and rhythm control) therapy.[44,60–67] Anselmino and colleagues[61] analyzed 26 observational studies, which included 1838 participants with AF (55% persistent) and HFrEF (mean EF 40%; 35% NYHA classes III and IV) to determine the efficacy of catheter ablation. After a mean follow-up of 23 months, freedom from atrial arrhythmia (atrial tachycardia lasting >30 seconds, atrial flutter, or AF after a 3-month blanking period) after a single procedure was 40%. The arrhythmia-free survival improved to 60% with multiple ablations. Ablations of complex fractionated electrograms and additional linear lesion ablations were performed in 54% and 45% of the patients, respectively.[61] An international multicenter registry, which enrolled 1273 patients with AF (65% persistent) who underwent catheter ablation, had a median follow-up of 3.6 years. No difference was noted in the number of AF ablations performed in patients with and without heart failure. The final procedural efficacy was 65% after a 3-month blanking period among patients with HFrEF.[60]

Multiple randomized controlled trials testing the efficacy of catheter ablation have demonstrated overall benefit compared with pharmacologic therapy (**Table 1**).[62–68] The only exception was the trial performed by MacDonald and colleagues[66]; 41 patients with HFrEF and persistent AF were randomized to catheter ablation versus medical therapy. No difference in N-terminal pro–brain natriuretic peptide level, LVEF, 6-minute walk distance, or quality of life was noted between both groups. However, 50% of the patients in this study who underwent catheter ablation remained in sinus rhythm at 6 months and had a complication rate of 15%.[66] Among the 7 randomized controlled trials, single-procedure efficacy ranged between 38% and 68%, and multiple-procedure efficacy ranged between 50% and 88% (**Fig. 1**). Among patients with recurrence of AF post–catheter ablation, a majority of the patients had significantly lower arrhythmia burden.[69,70] Long-term benefit, however, derived from reducing the burden of AF is currently unclear.

LVEF is an important surrogate outcome commonly tested in randomized controlled trials involving patients with HFrEF. Except for the trial by MacDonald and colleagues,[66] the rest of the randomized control trials have shown statistically significant improvement in LVEF with catheter ablation. It was previously believed that the improvement in LVEF is likely secondary to the restoration of sinus rhythm but not reflective of LV remodeling. The study by Di Baise and colleagues,[62] however, showed sustained improvement in LVEF up to 24 months from index procedure. Prabhu and colleagues[67] have shown that the absence of ventricular scar at baseline was associated with greater improvement in LVEF patients undergoing catheter ablation. This suggests that patients with ventricular scar are more susceptible to AF-induced cardiomyopathy. Therefore, this subgroup of patients may benefit with the restoration of normal sinus rhythm.

Exercise tolerance assessed by 6-minute walk test and peak oxygen consumption ($Vo_{2max}$) showed significant improvement in patients who underwent catheter ablation.[62–65] This was further tested by the authors' group in a meta-analysis which showed consistent benefit in exercise capacity with catheter ablation.[44] Quality of life assessed using the Minnesota Living with Heart Failure MLWHF showed significant benefit in patients who underwent catheter ablation. Patients enrolled the PABA-HF (Pulmonary Vein Antrum Isolation vs AV Node Ablation With Biventricular Pacing for Treatment of Atrial Fibrillation in Patients With Congestive Heart Failure) trial[63] had the highest preprocedural MLWHF scores and

**Table 1**
Characteristics of studies included in the systematic review

| Author | Population | Intervention | Comparator | Primary Outcome | Secondary Outcome | Time | Adverse Events |
|---|---|---|---|---|---|---|---|
| Khan et al,[63] 2008 | Persistent AF<br>EF ≤40%<br>NYHA II–III<br>N = 82 | CA<br>Isolation of PV<br>CFAE and linear lesions as per operator | AVN ablation + BiV pacing | Composite of<br>• EF<br>• 6MWD<br>• MLWHF score | • AF recurrence<br>• LA diameter<br>• QOL by MLWHF<br>• 6MWD<br>• HF readmission<br>• Change in EF | 12 mo | 3 groin bleeds<br>1 pericardial effusion<br>1 pulmonary edema<br>2 pulmonary vein stenoses<br>Control group<br>1 LV lead dislodgement<br>2 pocket hematomas<br>1 pneumothorax |
| MacDonald et al,[66] 2011 | Persistent AF<br>NYHA II–IV<br>EF ≤35%<br>N = 41 | CA<br>Isolation of PV<br>CFAE<br>Linear lines<br>CTI—case by case | Rate control | EF change by CMR | • NT BNP<br>• 6MWD<br>• QOL by MLWHF<br>• KCCQ<br>• AF recurrence<br>• HF readmission<br>• Change in EF | 6 mo | 1 patient stroke<br>2 tamponades<br>3 worsening HFs |
| Jones et al,[65] 2013 | Persistent AF<br>NYHA II–IV<br>EF ≤35%<br>N = 52 | CA<br>Isolation of PV<br>Linear lines<br>CFAE | Rate control | 12-mo change in $V_{O_{2max}}$ consumption | • QOL by MLWHF<br>• All-cause mortality<br>• BNP<br>• 6MWD<br>• EF<br>• AF recurrence<br>• HF readmission<br>• $V_{O_{2max}}$ | 12 mo | 1 pericardial effusion requiring sternotomy<br>2 temporary worsening HFs<br>1 groin bleed<br>1 pneumonia |
| Hunter et al,[64] 2014 | Persistent AF<br>NYHA II–IV<br>EF <50%<br>Adequate rate control<br>N = 50 | CA<br>Isolation PV<br>CFAE<br>Linear lines<br>CTI line | Medical rate control | EF change | • LVESV change<br>• All-cause mortality<br>• $V_{O_{2max}}$<br>• BNP<br>• NYHA class<br>• QOL by MLWHF<br>• SF-36<br>• AF recurrence<br>• Change in EF | 12 mo | 1 stroke<br>1 tamponade |

(continued on next page)

**Table 1**
*(continued)*

| Author | Population | Intervention | Comparator | Primary Outcome | Secondary Outcome | Time | Adverse Events |
|---|---|---|---|---|---|---|---|
| Di Biase et al,[62] 2016 | Persistent AF NYHA II–III EF <40% N = 203 | CA Isolation of PV Posterior wall SVC | Amiodarone + standard medical therapy (ACE/ARB, β-blockers, diuretics, digoxin) | AF recurrence | • HF readmission<br>• All-cause mortality<br>• Change in EF<br>• 6MWD<br>• QOL by MLWHF<br>• AF recurrence | 24 mo | 2 groin hematomas<br>1 pericardial effusion |
| Prabhu et al,[67] 2017 | Persistent AF Nonischemic NYHA II–IV EF ≤45% N = 36 | CA Isolation of PV Posterior wall | Medical rate control | Change in EF at 6 mo | • Chamber dimensions<br>• NYHA class<br>• BNP<br>• 6MWD<br>• SF 36 scores<br>• AF recurrence<br>• Change in EF | 6 mo | 4 unplanned admissions in the medical therapy arm<br>1 groin bleed<br>1 ILR bleed requiring transfusion |
| Marrouche et al,[68] 2018 | Paroxysmal or persistent AF NYHA II–IV EF ≤35% N = 363 | CA | Rate control | Composite<br>• Mortality<br>• HF admissions | • CVA<br>• All-cause mortality<br>• QOL<br>• 6MWD<br>• ICD therapies<br>• EF<br>• AF burden<br>• AF-free interval<br>• Time to ICD therapies<br>• HF readmission | 60 mo | 3 pericardial effusions<br>1 PV stenosis<br>3 acute bleeds<br>19 strokes (7 interventions and 12 controls)<br>4 pneumonias (3 interventions and 1 control)<br>1 groin infection<br>1 worsening CHF |

*Abbreviations:* 6MWD, 6-minute walk distance; ARB, angiotensin receptor blocker; AVN, atrioventricular node; BiV, biventricular; BNP, brain natriuretic peptide; CA, catheter ablation; CHF, congestive heart failure admission; CFAE, complex fractionated atrial electrograms; CMR, cardiac magnetic resonance; CTI, cavotricuspid isthmus; CV, cardiovascular; CVA, cerebrovascular accident; EF, ejection fraction; HF, heart failure; ILR, implantable loop recorder; KCCQ, Kansas City cardiomyopathy questionnaire; LA, left atrium; LVESV, left ventricular end-systolic volume; MLWHF, Minnesota living with heart failure; NT, N-terminal; PV, pulmonary veins; QOL, quality of life; SF-36, 36-item short form health survey; SVC, superior vena cava.

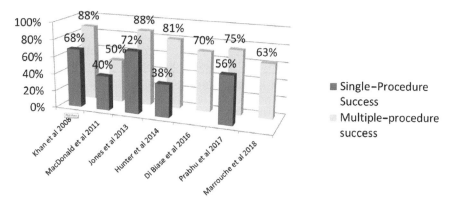

**Fig. 1.** Seven randomized controlled trials.

displayed the most improvement in MLWHF score compared with patients in other clinical trials. Improvement in quality-of-life metrics and exercise tolerance among the patients who undergo catheter ablation likely could be explained by a decrease in AF burden and improvement in LVEF.

Among the 7 randomized controlled trials, only CASTLE-AF trial[68] was powered to assess the mortality and hospitalization with catheter ablation. Patients with HFrEF with NYHA greater than class I, symptomatic persistent or paroxysmal AF (LVEF ≤35%), with implantable cardioverter defibrillator (ICD)/cardiac resynchronization therapy device (CRT-D) implantation were randomized to catheter ablation or medical therapy. A 16.1% absolute reduction in death or hospitalization was noted at 3 years (HR 0.62; 95% CI, 0.43–0.87; P = .006). In the authors' meta-analysis, statistically significant all-cause mortality benefit was demonstrated with catheter ablation in patients with AF and HFrEF (RR 0.52; 95% CI, 0.35–0.76; P = .001). Rate control with β-blockers was shown to have an incremental mortality benefit in patients with HFrEF in sinus rhythm, which was not seen in patients with persistent AF. This may suggest the benefit of rhythm control in patients with heart failure. The mortality benefit seen in the catheter ablation group also could be attributed to more patients in this group remaining in sinus rhythm compared with the control group. Moreover, in the past 5 years, the technology and modality of catheter ablation have dramatically changed. New advanced irrigated catheter tips and new modules, such as contact force monitoring systems, may have resulted in the relatively high success rate of catheter ablation for AF in HFrEF, which likely contributed to improvements in patient-centered outcomes.

Given the invasive nature of the procedure, catheter ablation carries certain procedural risk, including stroke, pericardial effusion, atrioesophageal fistula, bleeding, pulmonary stenosis,

pneumonia, and rarely death (see **Table 1**). The periprocedural complication rate in the authors' meta-analysis was 5.3%.[44] This was comparable to complication rates noted in prior studies (2.9%–5.2%) in patients with a structurally normal heart.[71,72] Most complications were related to postprocedural infections and access site bleeding. No procedural death was reported among the 7 randomized clinical trials.

## IMPACT OF CATHETER ABLATION IN HEART FAILURE WITH PRESERVED EJECTION FRACTION

In patients with HFpEF, AF confers a worse overall prognosis. In a recent meta-analysis of 20 studies on the impact of AF on all-cause mortality in heart failure, AF was associated with a poor prognosis in patients with HFpEF (random effects model pooled HR 1.21; 95% CI, 1.12–1.30) compared with patients with HFrEF (HR 1.09; 95% CI, 1.01–1.17).[73] Furthermore, the timing of AF and heart failure onset seems to have an impact on prognosis, where new-onset AF in prevalent HFpEF portends a worse prognosis regarding all-cause mortality compared with prevalent AF.[74] Compared with sinus rhythm, AF also has an impact on other patient-important outcomes in HFpEF, including greater exertion intolerance (10.8 mL/min/kg ± 3.1 mL/min/kg vs 13.5 mL/min/kg ± 3.8 mL/min/kg; P = .002; natriuretic peptide elevation (851–2637 pg/mL vs 272–1019 pg/mL; P<.0001); and greater left atrial volumes (57.8 mL/m$^2$ ± 17.0 mL/m$^2$ vs 42.5 mL/m$^2$ ± 15.1 mL/m$^2$; P = .001).[75] Unlike in HFrEF, where the benefit of ablation versus antiarrhythmic therapy is better characterized, the morbidity and mortality benefit of AF ablation in HFpEF are unclear.[62,68] One recent retrospective study investigated the difference in the effectiveness of AF ablation in HFpEF versus HFrEF and found no significant differences in arrhythmia-free recurrence or NYHA functional

**Table 2**
**Summary of ongoing trials on catheter ablation in patients with heart failure**

| Trial | Clinical Trial Identifier | Target Enrollment | Inclusion Criteria | Test Group | Control Group | Follow-up (mo) | Primary Outcomes |
|---|---|---|---|---|---|---|---|
| RAFT-AF | NCT01420393 | 600 | AF + BNP-positive HF (HFpEF and HFrEF) | Catheter ablation | Rate control | 24 | All-cause mortality and HF hospitalization |
| AFARC-LVF | NCT02509754 | 180 | Persistent AF + LVEF <35% | Catheter ablation | Rate control | 12 | Improvement in LVEF and NYHA class |
| CATCH-AF | NCT02686749 | 220 | AF + LVEF 25%–35% | Catheter ablation | Rate control | 12 | HF hospitalization and recurrent AF |
| AMICA | NCT00652522 | 216 | AF + ICD or CRT-D + LVEF <35% | Catheter ablation | Pharmacologic rate/rhythm control | 12 | LVEF by echocardiogram |

*Abbreviations:* BNP, brain natriuretic peptide; HF, heart failure; MR, mortality rate.

improvements between the 2 groups, suggesting that the benefits of ablation in HFrEF may apply to HFpEF.[76]

## CLINICAL IMPLICATIONS AND FUTURE DIRECTIONS

There is a growing body of evidence supporting the benefit of catheter ablation for AF in patients with HFrEF. Emphasis must be placed, however, on optimization of guideline-directed medical therapy for heart failure either during the blanking periods or in a run-in period. Otherwise, it could lead to overestimation of the benefit of catheter ablation. Currently, 4 ongoing randomized clinical trials are scheduled to be completed in 2019, which will further improve understanding of the utility catheter ablation in patients with HFrEF and AF (**Table 2**). The RAFT-AF (Resynchronization-Defibrillation for Ambulatory Heart Failure) trial (NCT01420393) is randomizing brain natriuretic peptide–confirmed HFrEF and HFpEF patients with AF to catheter ablation versus rate control strategy, with primary outcomes of interest all-cause mortality and HF hospitalization. The CATCH-AF (Catheter Ablation Versus Medical Therapy in Congested Hearts with AF) trial (NCT02686749) will test the efficacy of catheter ablation on recurrent heart failure hospitalization. Both AMICA (Atrial Fibrillation Management in Congestive Heart Failure With Ablation) (NCT00652522) and AFARC-LVF (Atrial Fibrillation

Ablation Compared to Rate Control Strategy in Patients With Impaired Left Ventricular Function) trials (NCT02509754) are enrolling patients with persistent AF and HFrEF. These trials hopefully will help identify the patient population who will benefit the most with catheter ablation.

## SUMMARY

Significant interplay between HFrEF and AF presents a therapeutic challenge for physicians. Given the efficacy and safety of catheter ablation in patients with HFrEF, there is increased use of catheter ablation as a treatment modality of choice, despite requiring multiple ablations to achieve long-term arrhythmia-free survival. Successful ablation of AF improved quality of life, LVEF, and exercise performance, as evidenced by improvement in MLWHF score, improved peak oxygen consumption, lower brain natriuretic peptide levels, and increased 6-minute walk distance. Cather ablation in patients with AF and HFrEF improves mortality and reduces heart failure hospitalizations. Future randomized controlled trials must focus on patients with HFpEF, given the lack of high-quality evidence in this population.

## REFERENCES

1. Kirchhof P, Benussi S, Kotecha D, et al. 2016 ESC guidelines for the management of atrial fibrillation developed in collaboration with EACTS. Europace 2016;18(11):1609–78.

2. Kishore A, Vail A, Majid A, et al. Detection of atrial fibrillation after ischemic stroke or transient ischemic attack: a systematic review and meta-analysis. Stroke 2014;45(2):520–6.

3. Sanna T, Diener HC, Passman RS, et al. Cryptogenic stroke and underlying atrial fibrillation. N Engl J Med 2014;370(26):2478–86.

4. Schnabel RB, Yin X, Gona P, et al. 50 year trends in atrial fibrillation prevalence, incidence, risk factors, and mortality in the Framingham Heart Study: a cohort study. Lancet 2015;386(9989):154–62.

5. Wang TJ, Larson MG, Levy D, et al. Temporal relations of atrial fibrillation and congestive heart failure and their joint influence on mortality: the Framingham Heart Study. Circulation 2003; 107(23):2920–5.

6. Braunwald E. Shattuck lecture–cardiovascular medicine at the turn of the millennium: triumphs, concerns, and opportunities. N Engl J Med 1997; 337(19):1360–9.

7. Kannel WB, Abbott RD, Savage DD, et al. Epidemiologic features of chronic atrial fibrillation: the Framingham study. N Engl J Med 1982;306(17):1018–22.

8. Benjamin EJ, Levy D, Vaziri SM, et al. Independent risk factors for atrial fibrillation in a population-based cohort. The Framingham Heart Study. JAMA 1994;271(11):840–4.

9. Maisel WH, Stevenson LW. Atrial fibrillation in heart failure: epidemiology, pathophysiology, and rationale for therapy. Am J Cardiol 2003;91(6a):2d–8d.

10. Bhatia RS, Tu JV, Lee DS, et al. Outcome of heart failure with preserved ejection fraction in a population-based study. N Engl J Med 2006; 355(3):260–9.

11. Owan TE, Hodge DO, Herges RM, et al. Trends in prevalence and outcome of heart failure with preserved ejection fraction. N Engl J Med 2006; 355(3):251–9.

12. Parkash R, Maisel WH, Toca FM, et al. Atrial fibrillation in heart failure: high mortality risk even if ventricular function is preserved. Am Heart J 2005;150(4):701–6.

13. Brignole M, Menozzi C, Gasparini M, et al. An evaluation of the strategy of maintenance of sinus rhythm by antiarrhythmic drug therapy after ablation and pacing therapy in patients with paroxysmal atrial fibrillation. Eur Heart J 2002;23(11): 892–900.

14. Carlsson J, Miketic S, Windeler J, et al. Randomized trial of rate-control versus rhythm-control in persistent atrial fibrillation: the Strategies of Treatment of Atrial Fibrillation (STAF) study. J Am Coll Cardiol 2003;41(10):1690–6.

15. Flaker GC, Blackshear JL, McBride R, et al. Antiarrhythmic drug therapy and cardiac mortality in atrial fibrillation. The Stroke Prevention in Atrial Fibrillation Investigators. J Am Coll Cardiol 1992; 20(3):527–32.

16. Hohnloser SH, Kuck KH, Lilienthal J. Rhythm or rate control in atrial fibrillation–Pharmacological Intervention in Atrial Fibrillation (PIAF): a randomised trial. Lancet 2000;356(9244):1789–94.

17. Roy D, Talajic M, Nattel S, et al. Rhythm control versus rate control for atrial fibrillation and heart failure. N Engl J Med 2008;358(25):2667–77.

18. Vorperian VR, Havighurst TC, Miller S, et al. Adverse effects of low dose amiodarone: a meta-analysis. J Am Coll Cardiol 1997;30(3):791–8.

19. Wyse DG, Waldo AL, DiMarco JP, et al. A comparison of rate control and rhythm control in patients with atrial fibrillation. N Engl J Med 2002;347(23):1825–33.

20. Clark DM, Plumb VJ, Epstein AE, et al. Hemodynamic effects of an irregular sequence of ventricular cycle lengths during atrial fibrillation. J Am Coll Cardiol 1997;30(4):1039–45.

21. Daoud EG, Weiss R, Bahu M, et al. Effect of an irregular ventricular rhythm on cardiac output. Am J Cardiol 1996;78(12):1433–6.

22. Rosca M, Lancellotti P, Popescu BA, et al. Left atrial function: pathophysiology, echocardiographic assessment, and clinical applications. Heart 2011; 97(23):1982–9.

23. Byrne M, Kaye DM, Power J. The synergism between atrial fibrillation and heart failure. J Card Fail 2008;14(4):320–6.

24. Tuinenburg AE, Van Veldhuisen DJ, Boomsma F, et al. Comparison of plasma neurohormones in congestive heart failure patients with atrial fibrillation versus patients with sinus rhythm. Am J Cardiol 1998;81(10):1207–10.

25. Wasmund SL, Li JM, Page RL, et al. Effect of atrial fibrillation and an irregular ventricular response on sympathetic nerve activity in human subjects. Circulation 2003;107(15):2011–5.

26. Gertz ZM, Raina A, Saghy L, et al. Evidence of atrial functional mitral regurgitation due to atrial fibrillation: reversal with arrhythmia control. J Am Coll Cardiol 2011;58(14):1474–81.

27. Dandamudi G, Rampurwala AY, Mahenthiran J, et al. Persistent left ventricular dilatation in tachycardia-induced cardiomyopathy patients after appropriate treatment and normalization of ejection fraction. Heart Rhythm 2008;5(8):1111–4.

28. Shinbane JS, Wood MA, Jensen DN, et al. Tachycardia-induced cardiomyopathy: a review of animal models and clinical studies. J Am Coll Cardiol 1997;29(4):709–15.

29. Van Gelder IC, Crijns HJ, Blanksma PK, et al. Time course of hemodynamic changes and improvement of exercise tolerance after cardioversion of chronic atrial fibrillation unassociated with cardiac valve disease. Am J Cardiol 1993;72(7):560–6.

30. Fenelon G, Wijns W, Andries E, et al. Tachycardiomyopathy: mechanisms and clinical implications. Pacing Clin Electrophysiol 1996;19(1):95–106.

31. McCullough PA, Philbin EF, Spertus JA, et al. Confirmation of a heart failure epidemic: findings from the resource utilization among congestive heart failure (REACH) study. J Am Coll Cardiol 2002;39(1):60–9.

32. Hunter RJ, Liu Y, Lu Y, et al. Left atrial wall stress distribution and its relationship to electrophysiologic remodeling in persistent atrial fibrillation. Circ Arrhythm Electrophysiol 2012;5(2):351–60.

33. Caldeira D, David C, Sampaio C. Rate versus rhythm control in atrial fibrillation and clinical outcomes: updated systematic review and meta-analysis of randomized controlled trials. Arch Cardiovasc Dis 2012;105(4):226–38.

34. Wyse D. Atrial Fibrillation Follow-up Investigation of Rhythm Management (AFFIRM) Investigators: a comparison of rate control and rhythm control in patients with atrial fibrillation. N Engl J Med 2002;347: 1825–33.

35. January CT, Wann LS, Alpert JS, et al. 2014 AHA/ACC/HRS guideline for the management of patients with atrial fibrillation: a report of the American College of Cardiology/American Heart Association Task Force on practice guidelines and the heart rhythm society. J Am Coll Cardiol 2014;64(21): e1–76.

36. Køber L, Torp-Pedersen C, McMurray JJ, et al. Increased mortality after dronedarone therapy for severe heart failure. N Engl J Med 2008;358(25): 2678–87.

37. Torp-Pedersen C, Møller M, Bloch-Thomsen PE, et al. Dofetilide in patients with congestive heart failure and left ventricular dysfunction. N Engl J Med 1999;341(12):857–65.

38. Brendorp B, Elming H, Jun L, et al. QTc interval as a guide to select those patients with congestive heart failure and reduced left ventricular systolic function who will benefit from antiarrhythmic treatment with dofetilide. Circulation 2001;103(10): 1422–7.

39. Rienstra M, Damman K, Mulder BA, et al. Beta-blockers and outcome in heart failure and atrial fibrillation: a meta-analysis. JACC Heart Fail 2013; 1(1):21–8.

40. Cullington D, Goode KM, Zhang J, et al. Is heart rate important for patients with heart failure in atrial fibrillation? JACC Heart Fail 2014;2(3):213–20.

41. Kotecha D, Flather MD, Altman DG, et al. Heart rate and rhythm and the benefit of beta-blockers in patients with heart failure. J Am Coll Cardiol 2017; 69(24):2885–96.

42. Kotecha D, Holmes J, Krum H, et al. Efficacy of β blockers in patients with heart failure plus atrial fibrillation: an individual-patient data meta-analysis. Lancet 2014;384(9961):2235–43.

43. Pedersen OD, Bagger H, Keller N, et al. Efficacy of dofetilide in the treatment of atrial fibrillation-flutter in patients with reduced left ventricular function: a

Danish investigations of arrhythmia and mortality on dofetilide (diamond) substudy. Circulation 2001; 104(3):292–6.

44. Agasthi P, Lee JZ, Amin M, et al. Catheter ablation for treatment of atrial fibrillation in patients with heart failure with reduced ejection fraction: a systematic review and meta-analysis. J Arrhythmia 2019.

45. Elgendy AY, Mahmoud AN, Khan MS, et al. Meta-analysis comparing catheter-guided ablation versus conventional medical therapy for patients with atrial fibrillation and heart failure with reduced ejection fraction. Am J Cardiol 2018;122(5): 806–13.

46. Khan SU, Rahman H, Talluri S, et al. The clinical benefits and mortality reduction associated with catheter ablation in subjects with atrial fibrillation: a systematic review and meta-analysis. JACC Clin Electrophysiol 2018;4(5):626–35.

47. Calkins H, Hindricks G, Cappato R, et al. 2017 HRS/EHRA/ECAS/APHRS/SOLAECE expert consensus statement on catheter and surgical ablation of atrial Heart Rhythm 2017;14(10):e275–444.

48. Berntsen RF, Håland TF, Skårdal R, et al. Focal impulse and rotor modulation as a stand-alone procedure for the treatment of paroxysmal atrial fibrillation: a within-patient controlled study with implanted cardiac monitoring. Heart Rhythm 2016 13(9):1768–74.

49. Buch E, Share M, Tung R, et al. Long-term clinical outcomes of focal impulse and rotor modulation for treatment of atrial fibrillation: a multicenter experience. Heart Rhythm 2016;13(3):636–41.

50. Cutler MJ, Johnson J, Abozguia K, et al. Impact of voltage mapping to guide whether to perform ablation of the posterior wall in patients with persistent atrial fibrillation. J Cardiovasc Electrophysiol 2016 27(1):13–21.

51. Fink T, Schlüter M, Heeger C-H, et al. Stand-alone pulmonary vein isolation versus pulmonary vein isolation with additional substrate modification as index ablation procedures in patients with persistent and long-standing persistent atrial fibrillation: the Randomized Alster-Lost-AF Trial (Ablation at St Georg Hospital for Long-Standing Persistent Atrial Fibrillation). Circ Arrhythm Electrophysiol 2017 10(7):e005114.

52. Jadidi AS, Lehrmann H, Keyl C, et al. Ablation of persistent atrial fibrillation targeting low-voltage areas with selective activation characteristics. Circ Arrhythm Electrophysiol 2016;9(3):e002962.

53. Miller JM, Kalra V, Das MK, et al. Clinical benefit of ablating localized sources for human atrial fibrillation: the Indiana University FIRM Registry. J Am Coll Cardiol 2017;69(10):1247–56.

54. Nery PB, Thornhill R, Nair GM, et al. Scar-based catheter ablation for persistent atrial fibrillation Curr Opin Cardiol 2017;32(1):1–9.

55. Oral H, Chugh A, Good E, et al. A tailored approach to catheter ablation of paroxysmal atrial fibrillation. Circulation 2006;113(15):1824–31.

56. Zhao Y, Di Biase L, Trivedi C, et al. Importance of non–pulmonary vein triggers ablation to achieve long-term freedom from paroxysmal atrial fibrillation in patients with low ejection fraction. Heart Rhythm 2016;13(1):141–9.

57. Nery PB, Belliveau D, Nair GM, et al. Relationship between pulmonary vein reconnection and atrial fibrillation recurrence: a systematic review and meta-analysis. JACC Clin Electrophysiol 2016;2(4):474–83.

58. Parikh SS, Jons C, McNitt S, et al. Predictive capability of left atrial size measured by CT, TEE, and TTE for recurrence of atrial fibrillation following radiofrequency catheter ablation. Pacing Clin Electrophysiol 2010;33(5):532–40.

59. Tops LF, Bax JJ, Zeppenfeld K, et al. Effect of radiofrequency catheter ablation for atrial fibrillation on left atrial cavity size. Am J Cardiol 2006;97(8):1220–2.

60. Ullah W, Ling L-H, Prabhu S, et al. Catheter ablation of atrial fibrillation in patients with heart failure: impact of maintaining sinus rhythm on heart failure status and long-term rates of stroke and death. Europace 2016;18(5):679–86.

61. Anselmino M, Matta M, D'Ascenzo F, et al. Catheter ablation of atrial fibrillation in patients with left ventricular systolic dysfunction: a systematic review and meta-analysis. Circ Arrhythm Electrophysiol 2014;7(6):1011–8.

62. Di Biase L, Mohanty P, Mohanty S, et al. Ablation versus amiodarone for treatment of persistent atrial fibrillation in patients with congestive heart failure and an implanted device: results from the AATAC Multicenter Randomized Trial. Circulation 2016;133(17):1637–44.

63. Khan MN, Jais P, Cummings J, et al. Pulmonary-vein isolation for atrial fibrillation in patients with heart failure. N Engl J Med 2008;359(17):1778–85.

64. Hunter RJ, Berriman TJ, Diab I, et al. A randomized controlled trial of catheter ablation versus medical treatment of atrial fibrillation in heart failure (the CAMTAF trial). Circ Arrhythm Electrophysiol 2014;7(1):31–8.

65. Jones DG, Haldar SK, Hussain W, et al. A randomized trial to assess catheter ablation versus rate control in the management of persistent atrial fibrillation in heart failure. J Am Coll Cardiol 2013;61(18):1894–903.

66. MacDonald MR, Connelly DT, Hawkins NM, et al. Radiofrequency ablation for persistent atrial fibrillation in patients with advanced heart failure and severe left ventricular systolic dysfunction: a randomised controlled trial. Heart 2011;97(9):740–7.

67. Prabhu S, Taylor AJ, Costello BT, et al. Catheter ablation versus medical rate control in atrial fibrillation and systolic dysfunction: the CAMERA-MRI study. J Am Coll Cardiol 2017;70(16):1949–61.

68. Marrouche NF, Brachmann J, Andresen D, et al. Catheter ablation for atrial fibrillation with heart failure. N Engl J Med 2018;378(5):417–27.

69. Oral H, Pappone C, Chugh A, et al. Circumferential pulmonary-vein ablation for chronic atrial fibrillation. N Engl J Med 2006;354(9):934–41.

70. Verma A, Champagne J, Sapp J, et al. Discerning the incidence of symptomatic and asymptomatic episodes of atrial fibrillation before and after catheter ablation (DISCERN AF): a prospective, multicenter study. JAMA Intern Med 2013;173(2):149–56.

71. Bohnen M, Stevenson WG, Tedrow UB, et al. Incidence and predictors of major complications from contemporary catheter ablation to treat cardiac arrhythmias. Heart Rhythm 2011;8(11):1661–6.

72. Gupta A, Perera T, Ganesan A, et al. Complications of catheter ablation of atrial fibrillation: a systematic review. Circ Arrhythm Electrophysiol 2013;6(6):1082–8.

73. Cheng M, Lu X, Huang J, et al. The prognostic significance of atrial fibrillation in heart failure with a preserved and reduced left ventricular function: insights from a meta-analysis. Eur J Heart Fail 2014;16(12):1317–22.

74. Santhanakrishnan R, Wang N, Larson MG, et al. Atrial fibrillation begets heart failure and vice versa: temporal associations and differences in preserved versus reduced ejection fraction. Circulation 2016;133(5):484–92.

75. Lam CS, Rienstra M, Tay WT, et al. Atrial fibrillation in heart failure with preserved ejection fraction: association with exercise capacity, left ventricular filling pressures, natriuretic peptides, and left atrial volume. JACC Heart Fail 2017;5(2):92–8.

76. Black-Maier E, Ren X, Steinberg BA, et al. Catheter ablation of atrial fibrillation in patients with heart failure and preserved ejection fraction. Heart Rhythm 2018;15(5):651–7.

# Atrial Fibrillation Ablation Should Be First-Line Therapy in Heart Failure Patients: CON

Amanulla Khaji, MD[a],*, Colleen Hanley, MD[a],
Peter R. Kowey, MD, FHRS[b]

## KEYWORDS

- Atrial fibrillation • Heart failure with reduced ejection fraction
- Heart failure with preserved ejection fraction • Catheter ablation
- Cardiac resynchronization therapy

## KEY POINTS

- Atrial fibrillation (AF) and heart failure are common cardiac conditions that often coexist, due to common risk factors and a complex interplay of the pathophysiology of these 2 disease entities.
- AF and heart failure share common disease mechanisms and treatment strategies.
- Optimal medical management of heart failure may protect against the occurrence of AF and therapies targeting AF may prevent the development of congestive heart failure.
- It is important to stress that effective treatment of AF may be achieved only with the simultaneous treatment of heart failure, and vice versa: satisfactory management of AF is essential for the optimum treatment of heart failure.

## BACKGROUND

Heart failure (HF) and atrial fibrillation (AF) have become epidemics of the twenty-first century, in part due to increased longevity and the success in reducing overall cardiovascular (CV) mortality.[1] Chronic HF is a highly prevalent disorder, afflicting approximately 6 million individuals in the United States, with an incidence of 10 in 1000 persons older than 65 years.[2] AF, like HF, affects millions of patients and markedly increases in prevalence with age. There is a sinister synergism between AF and HF. These common cardiovascular conditions often coexist and result in significant morbidity and mortality. Despite the extensive amount of research and literature about each of these disorders separately, randomized controlled clinical trial data concerning the management of AF in patients with HF is lacking. Given the poor outcomes associated with HF and AF, finding effective therapies for these patients is of paramount importance but remains a challenge. Treatment of AF has progressed over past 2 decades; however, unanswered questions remain, most importantly, what is the best treatment strategy? In this article, we provide an in-depth review of the management of AF in patients with HF and provide insight as to why catheter ablation should not be the first line of therapy in this population.

Disclosure: Dr P.R. Kowey served on the steering committee of the CABANA trial. Drs A. Khaji and C. Hanley have nothing to disclose.
[a] Lankenau Heart Institute, 100 East Lancaster Avenue, Wynnewood, PA 19087, USA; [b] Lankenau Heart Institute, Jefferson Medical College, 111 S 11th Street, Philadelphia, PA 19107, USA
* Corresponding author.
E-mail address: khajia@gmail.com

## Epidemiology

Nearly 300,000 Americans die from HF annually, and although overall survival has improved over time, mortality remains high, as roughly 50% of patients die within 5 years of diagnosis.[3] HF is the strongest predictor for the development of AF, with up to a sixfold increase in risk seen in the Framingham Study.[4] AF is the most common arrhythmia, with an estimated prevalence in the United States ranging from 2.7 to 6.1 million in 2010 and a projected increase in its prevalence over time. As the population ages globally, AF is predicted to affect 6 to 12 million people in the United States by 2050 and 17.9 million in Europe by 2060.[5–7] More recent HF series report a prevalence of AF ranging from 13% to 27%, and the prevalence of AF increases in parallel with the degree of heart failure. Patients with New York Heart Association (NYHA) functional class I have an AF prevalence of less than 5%, whereas those with NYHA functional class IV symptoms have a prevalence of AF up to 50%.[8] In all, 15% to 20% of patients with HF are in AF at first evaluation,[9] whereas 27% to 48% of patients who undergo cardioversion of AF demonstrate a symptomatology of NYHA class III-IV heart failure.[10] The prevalence of AF in patients with heart failure with preserved systolic function (HFpEF) is less well-established. Both these conditions are associated with older age, hypertension, and diastolic dysfunction; therefore, these disorders are inextricably linked, both to each other and to adverse cardiovascular outcomes. Surveys, registries, and trials have given insight into the prevalence of HFpEF in patients with AF, which varies between 8% and 24%,[11–14] and depends on the definition of HFpEF (left ventricular ejection fraction [LVEF] above 40% or 50%) and the type of AF.

## PATHOPHYSIOLOGY

HF is characterized by hemodynamic changes that increase the pressure and the volume of the atria and lead to disturbances of atrial electrical properties favoring the development of AF. Under normal circumstances, atrial systole may contribute up to 25% of the cardiac output. In the setting of ventricular dysfunction, the atrial contribution to the total cardiac output could be as high as 50%. The onset of AF abolishes the "atrial kick" leading to reductions in cardiac output, peak oxygen uptake, and exercise tolerance.[15] When the failing heart is subjected to these adverse hemodynamic conditions, cardiac decompensation occurs.

The onset of AF also decreases cardiac output and worsens HF through additional mechanisms.

AF may lead to more pronounced valvular regurgitation, which causes reduction in forward blood flow. Rapid ventricular rates during periods of uncontrolled AF lead to inadequate ventricle filling time and decrease in stroke volume.[16–18] An irregular ventricular response, in itself and independent of heart rate, causes a drop in cardiac output, increase in pulmonary wedge pressure, and elevation of right atrial pressure.[19] In patients with normal baseline ventricular function, chronic rapid ventricular rates associated with AF can lead to tachycardia-induced cardiomyopathy.

Ultrastructural cardiac remodeling occurs, characterized by cytoskeletal alteration, matrix metalloproteinase disruption, depletion of high-energy stores, and induction of abnormal calcium handling. The negative remodeling process is also accompanied by neurohormonal derangements, such as increased sympathetic response and activation of the renin-angiotensin system (RAS).[20–22]

High intracardiac volumes and pressures in HF can cause mechanical stretching of the atria, which is associated with shortening of the atrial refractory period, prolongation of atrial conduction times, increased frequency of interatrial conduction blocks, and heightened atrial irritability.[23,24] Stimulation of the sympathetic nervous system and high catecholamine levels that are features of chronic HF not only increase the ventricular rate response in AF, but may cause abnormalities of atrial action potentials and automaticity that can trigger arrhythmogenesis as well.[25] Parasympathetic hyper innervation is part of a complex autonomic remodeling process seen in HF, and contributes significantly to the maintenance of AF.[26] Activation of the RAS system in HF leads to increased angiotensin-II expression, which induces atrial interstitial fibrosis, creating areas of slowed conduction and heterogeneity in repolarization that serve as substrates for AF generation.[2] In the failing atrium, profound calcium dysregulation and ion channel remodeling within the atrial cardiomyocyte enhance arrhythmogenesis and promote triggered activity in AF.[28]

At a molecular level, abnormal distribution of gap junctions and loss of cell-to-cell coupling in areas of fibrosis contribute to electrical remodeling, increased (and dispersed) atrial refractoriness and development of AF.[29,30] Disrupted ion channel regulation has been demonstrated in experimental models of HF, with reduction in the L-type calcium ion ($Ca^{2+}$) current, the sensitive transient outward potassium ion ($K^+$) current and the slow delayed rectifier $K^+$ current in atrial myocytes,[31] whereas the transient inward sodium ion ($Na^+$)/$Ca^{2+}$ exchanger current is increased.[3]

The increase in the $Na^+/Ca2^+$ transmembrane exchange channel current gives rise to delayed afterdepolarizations, leading to arrhythmias initiated by triggered activity.[28] The important role of gap junctions in atrial remodeling has also been highlighted, involving atrial connexin proteins[33–38] and the resultant inhomogeneity of impulse propagation, thus establishing the substrate for reentrant circuits and AF.

## MEDICAL THERAPY OF PATIENTS WITH ATRIAL FIBRILLATION AND HEART FAILURE
### Rate Control

Patients with HF who develop AF have an increased morbidity and mortality, which would suggest that the restoration and maintenance of sinus rhythm in these patients might improve their long-term outcomes. However, there are currently no data to support that pursuing a rhythm control strategy provides any major benefit over rate control. There are several reasons that rhythm control has failed to improve survival in clinical trials, including limited efficacy and adverse effects of available treatments, or delayed intervention such that the cumulative effects of AF are already unable to be reversed. Sinus rhythm can be difficult to achieve and maintain, particularly in patients with HF.

Beta-blockers are a mainstay in the treatment of HF with reduced ejection fraction (HFrEF). Numerous randomized clinical trials have shown a substantial reduction in all-cause mortality, CV death, and hospitalization compared with placebo. In these trials, between 8% and 23% of enrolled participants were in AF at baseline.[39] Pooling individual patient data from 11 randomized controlled trials (with 96% of recruited participants ever enrolled in such trials), the adjusted hazard ratio (HR) for all-cause mortality for beta-blockers versus placebo was 0.73 (95% confidence interval [CI] 0.67–0.80) in sinus rhythm. In patients with AF, the HR was 0.97 (95% CI 0.83–1.14). The lack of benefit in AF was consistent across all subgroups, including age categories, gender, NYHA class, and baseline heart rate; however, their use is widespread for control of heart rate in AF, both acutely and for long-term management. In the acute setting of HF with rapid AF, beta-blockers are useful for rate-reduction and preferred to digoxin due to their effectiveness at high sympathetic tone. For long-term control of heart rate, beta-blockers are traditionally the first-line choice for clinicians.

There has been a decline in the use of the cardiac glycoside, digoxin, following the DIG trial, which showed no mortality benefit with the use of digoxin in patients with HF with sinus rhythm.[40,41] In observational studies and post hoc analysis of randomized clinical trials, there have been concerns about increased mortality with digoxin,[42] but equally a number of studies have found no association.[43–46] There are currently no direct randomized comparisons of digoxin use in patients with AF. Digoxin should be used cautiously in appropriate patients, with no expectation of effect on mortality.

### Antiarrhythmic Drug Therapy

The choice of antiarrhythmic drug options is limited in patients with HF due to potential proarrhythmia and/or negative inotropy. The use of class IC agents was associated with increased mortality in the Cardiac Arrhythmia Suppression Trial (CAST) in patients with ventricular ectopy after myocardial infarction, and their use is not recommended in patients with structural heart disease.[47] Dronedarone is a derivative of amiodarone with a shorter half-life and is devoid of iodine moiety to reduce toxicity. It was studied in the Antiarrhythmic Trial with Dronedarone in Moderate to Severe CHF Evaluating Morbidity Decrease (ANDROMEDA) trial,[48] in patients with advanced HF and AF. ANDROMEDA found a twofold excess in mortality with dronedarone compared with placebo, primarily due to worsening HF, prompting the early termination of this study after just 2 months of clinical follow-up. As a result, dronedarone carries a black box warning listing severely symptomatic or recently decompensated HF as a contraindication.

Of the available antiarrhythmic drugs, only amiodarone and dofetilide have been shown not to increase mortality in patients with HF.[49,50] In the DIAMOND study, patients were randomized to dofetilide versus placebo. The probability of maintaining sinus rhythm for 1 year was 79% with dofetilide versus 42% with placebo. Although dofetilide had no effect on all-cause mortality, restoration and maintenance of sinus rhythm was associated with significant reduction in mortality (risk ratio [RR] 0.44; 95% CI 0.30–0.64; $P<.0001$). In addition, dofetilide therapy was associated with a significantly lower RR versus placebo rehospitalization.[51] Similar conclusions were reached in the CHF-STAT study, in which the mortality of patients who converted to sinus rhythm on amiodarone was significantly lower than in those who did not.[52]

## DEVICE-BASED THERAPY
### Cardiac Resynchronization Therapy and Atrioventricular Node Ablation

The major randomized controlled trials that demonstrated the efficacy of cardiac resynchronization therapy (CRT) excluded patients with AF. Yet, AF occurs in 1 of 4 recipients of CRT.[53,54] The prognosis of patients with AF with CRT is worse than that of patients in sinus rhythm.[55,56] They are at a major disadvantage due to loss of atrioventricular (AV) synchronicity, insufficient CRT delivery as a result of uncontrolled ventricular rates, higher rates of appropriate implantable cardioverter defibrillator (ICD) shocks for ventricular arrhythmia as well as inappropriate ICD shocks. Consequently, patients with CRT and AF have inadequate symptomatic improvement, repeated hospitalization, and increased mortality.[57] Furthermore, AF is associated with fusion and pseudo-fusion, which represents inefficient biventricular capture. Such beats render the pacing counters inaccurate for assessing true biventricular capture beats. AF represents an important cause of poor long-term CRT benefit and prognosis unless aggressive efforts are made to slow the ventricular rate.[58]

The results of the Resynchronization for Ambulatory Heart Failure Trial (RAFT AF) study were published in 2012.[59] This constitutes to date the largest, randomized report examining the role of CRT in patients with permanent AF. Although it showed no clear reduction in clinical events or improvement in objective surrogate measures, there was a trend favoring a reduction in HF hospitalizations with CRT-ICD. There was also a clear indication that CRT was suboptimally delivered; only one-third of patients received greater than 95% ventricular pacing. Again, even this may be an overestimate; Holter monitoring studies have shown that, when device logs indicate ≥90% ventricular pacing in patients with permanent AF without AV junction ablation, 53% of these paced beats are actually fusion or pseudo-fusion.

Many reports have emphasized that the control of the ventricular rate with AV blocking drugs is difficult and often yield suboptimal results. AV junctional ablation should be considered in all CRT patients in AF with rapid ventricular rate despite maximally tolerated doses of AV nodal blocking agents. AV junctional ablation permits CRT delivery close to 100% of the time with regularization of the RR intervals and elimination of fusion and pseudo-fusion beats. Patients who have undergone AV junctional ablation derive as much benefit from CRT as patients in sinus rhythm, provided the ventricular rate is controlled by AV junctional ablation. The CERTIFY trial was conducted to determine whether CRT confers similar benefits for patients with AF with or without AV junctional ablation.[60] The results of the CERTIFY trial demonstrated that in CRT patients with AF, AV junctional ablation is associated with a reduction in all-cause mortality, compared with rate-slowing drugs.

The more recently published APAF-CRT trial was a prospective, randomized, parallel, open-label clinical trial involving patients with severely symptomatic permanent AF and narrow QRS that compared pharmacologic rate control with AV junction ablation and CRT.[61] The primary composite outcome of death due to HF, or hospitalization due to HF, or worsening HF had occurred in 20% of patients in the Ablation plus CRT arm and in 38% in the Drug arm (HR 0.38; 95% CI 0.18–0.81; $P = .013$). Although this is a small, unblinded trial, it showed AV junction ablation and CRT is both safe and superior to conventional medical strategy in relieving symptoms of HF and reducing hospitalization for HF in patients affected by permanent AF despite a narrow QRS. Therefore, AV junction ablation and CRT is a reasonable option for patients with HF and AF. Accordingly, the American College of Cardiology/American Heart Association/Heart Rhythm Society guidelines indicate that CRT can be useful in patients with AF and LVEF less than or equal to 35% on guideline-directed medical therapy if the patient requires ventricular pacing or otherwise meets CRT criteria and AV nodal ablation or pharmacologic rate control will allow near 100% ventricular pacing with CRT (Level of Evidence: B).[62,63]

## CATHETER ABLATION

Our ever-expanding understanding of the mechanisms of AF and rapidly advancing technologies have made catheter-based ablation of AF an increasingly effective and safe treatment modality for rhythm control. It has become an established option for symptomatic AF that is resistant to drug therapy in patients with otherwise normal cardiac function.

### Current Guidelines on the Role of Catheter Ablation in Atrial Fibrillation

The current American and European guidelines for AF management do not make specific recommendations for patients with coexisting AF and HFrEF. In patients who have coexisting AF and HF, the main aims of treatment are to prevent adverse outcomes, improve symptoms, and maintain a good quality of life. The 2016 European Society guidelines on the management of AF state that the "indications for catheter ablation in HF patients with reduced ejection fraction (HFrEF) should be carefully balanced and procedures performed in experienced centers."[64] The guidelines also recognize that AF ablation can be more demanding in this patient cohort compared with patients without HF. In patients presenting acutely with AF and HF, the guidelines recommend focusing on normalizing fluid balance, aiming for an initial heart rate target of less than 110 beats per minute, use of anticoagulation, inhibition of the renin–angiotensin–aldosterone system and early consideration of rhythm control. The 2017 Heart Rhythm Society/European Heart Rhythm Association/European Cardiac Arrhythmia Society/Asia Pacific Heart Rhythm Society/Latin American Society of Cardiac Stimulation and Electrophysiology expert consensus statement on AF ablation recommends that it is reasonable to use similar indications for AF ablation in selected patients with HF as for patients without HF (class IIa, level of evidence B-R).[65] The optimal ablation strategy for patients with HFrEF remains controversial (**Fig 1**).

However, there is no clear consensus on which patients with HF should be offered catheter ablation or the optimal ablation strategy in this setting. A growing number of studies have now been published to assess the effectiveness of catheter ablation on improving clinical outcomes in patients with AF and HF. These studies have challenged previous treatment paradigms in which rate control was considered equivalent to rhythm control in this patient population.

There have been numerous retrospective observational studies examining outcomes of catheter ablation for AF in patients with HFrEF.[66] Despite showing safety and a trend toward improvement in left ventricular function and improved quality of life, these studies were single-center experiences and many were relatively small (<100 patients) sample sizes.

## Randomized Clinical Trials

Recently several randomized trials that have assessed the role of catheter ablation of AF in patients with CHF. These trials are summarized in. The Pulmonary Vein Antrum Isolation versus Atrioventricular Node Ablation with Biventricular Pacing for Treatment of Atrial Fibrillation in Patients with Congestive Heart Failure (PABA-CHF) trial[67] compared pulmonary vein isolation (n = 41) with AV node ablation plus biventricular pacing (n = 40) for the composite of ejection fraction, 6-minute walk distance, and Minnesota Living With Heart Failure (MLWHF) questionnaire.[25] The study showed pulmonary vein isolation to be superior to AV node ablation and biventricular pacing with

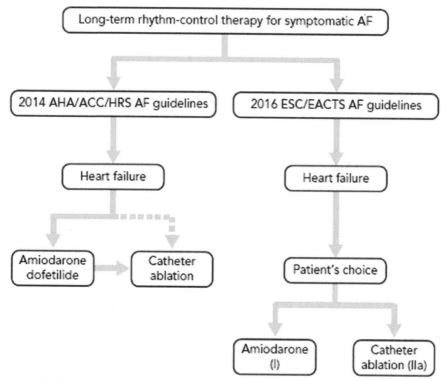

**Fig. 1.** Current guidelines for management of AF. ACC, American College of Cardiology; AHA, American Heart Association; EACTS, European Association for Cardio-Thoracic Surgery; ESC, European Society of Cardiology; HRS, Heart Rhythm Society. (*From* Packer DL, Mark DB, Robb RA, et al. Catheter ablation versus antiarrhythmic drug therapy for atrial fibrillation (CABANA) trial: study rationale and design. Am Heart J 2018;199:192–9; with permission.)

respect to the primary endpoint (composite of composite of ejection fraction, distance on the 6-minute walk test, and MLWHF score) but only followed patients for 6 months.

In the Ablation versus Amiodarone for Treatment of Persistent Atrial Fibrillation in Patients with Congestive Heart Failure and an Implanted Device (AATAC) trial, Di Biase and colleagues[68] randomized 203 patients with persistent AF, dual-chamber or biventricular ICD, and HFrEF to ablation versus amiodarone. The primary endpoint was AF recurrence and secondary endpoints were all-cause mortality and unplanned hospitalizations. Despite a wide range of single-procedure success rates between centers (29%–61%), those randomized to ablation were more likely to be in sinus rhythm after single and multiple procedures. Over 2 years of follow-up, the ablation group had lower rates of hospitalization (31% vs 57%, P<.001) and mortality (8% vs 18%, P = .037) compared with those randomized to amiodarone. However, this trial was not designed to assess clinical outcomes (hospitalization for HF, mortality). Results suggesting improved outcomes with AF ablation thus require validation. There are some limitations that should be kept in mind when considering the AATAC results. There was no rate-control arm and this prevents comparison of AF ablation (or anti arrhythmic drug therapy use) with what is considered standard of care in this population. In addition, multiple ablation procedures were allowed in the ablation arm (average of 1.4 procedures per patient) and there was no clear protocol for determining when a repeat procedure was indicated.

As shown in, the CAMERA-MRI and catheter ablation versus medical treatment of atrial fibrillation in heart failure (CAMTAF) trials showed trend toward benefit in the ablation arms. The CAMERA-MRI and CAMTAF trial both found that restoration of sinus rhythm with catheter ablation in patients with HF and AF improved important surrogate outcomes.[69,70] However, only a small number of patients were included in these trials, follow-up was limited to 1 year, and hard outcomes, such as mortality, were not examined.

Of all the randomized trials done in the past decade, only the Catheter Ablation versus Standard Conventional Therapy in Patients with Left Ventricular Dysfunction and Atrial Fibrillation (CASTLE AF) trial was prospectively designed and powered to examine hard outcomes in this specific population.[71] The trial included 397 patients with symptomatic paroxysmal or persistent AF, symptomatic HF, and LVEF of ≤35%

who were randomized to receive either radiofrequency catheter ablation or conventional drug therapy. All patients had an ICD with home monitoring capability. The primary endpoint was the composite of all-cause mortality or unplanned hospitalization for worsening HF. The results were trumpeted as proving beyond doubt that ablation should be used wholesale in patients with HF; however, there were important limitations to consider. The study recruited patients over a long period of time, screening more than 3000 to enroll only 397. With a small number of events in an open-labeled study, it is difficult to interpret the conclusions of the study. The reported benefits on LVEF and exercise tolerance were in a small number of patients and were typically nonsustained. Ablation reduced, but did not eliminate, episodes of AF: 63% of the ablation group versus 22% of the medical therapy group were in sinus rhythm at 60 months. The persistence of AF and the harmful effect of antiarrhythmic drug therapy in so many patients in the CASTLE trial might explain why, in APAF-CRT, they achieved an even greater reduction in the combined endpoint of death from any cause and hospitalization, with an HR of 0.26. However, the 2 trials cannot be directly compared, owing to major differences in baseline clinical characteristics. For example, CASTLE patients were, on average, 8 years younger, no patient was older than 71 years, 72% had intermittent AF, and 69% were in NYHA Class I or II. CASTLE AF does not apply to sicker, older, and frailer patients with HF. In a subgroup analysis, patients with an ejection fraction less than 25% showed a trend toward worse outcomes with ablation.

The results of recently published Catheter ABlation vs ANtiarrhythmic. Drug Therapy in Atrial Fibrillation (CABANA) trial are noteworthy to reflect the effect of AF ablation on hard outcomes.[72,73] The CABANA trial was a multicenter randomized controlled trial comparing catheter ablation with optimal medical therapy in patients with all forms of AF (paroxysmal, persistent, and longstanding persistent). This failed to show superiority of AF ablation for hard outcomes including all-cause mortality in patients with AF. A subgroup analysis in patients who had HF (only 15% in this study) by treatment actually received, had a significant 49% relative risk reduction with ablation and those with NYHA class II or worse HF had a significant 41% relative advantage with the procedure. This analysis was criticized because it was not intention to treat and because the primary endpoint was not reached in the overall primary analysis. Thus, the on treatment results in this subgroup should be considered only exploratory.

## SUMMARY

AF and HF are common cardiac conditions that often coexist, due to common risk factors and a complex interplay of the pathophysiology of these 2 disease entities. Their joint association correlates with adverse outcomes. AF and HF share common disease mechanisms and treatment strategies. Optimal medical management of heart failure may protect against the occurrence of AF and therapies targeting AF may prevent the development of congestive HF. The debate between a rate control and rhythm control strategy is now fueled with new studies exploring the role of catheter ablation. Based on results of completed clinical trials of AF ablation in HF, patients who tend to have the least benefit from catheter ablation appear to have a higher NYHA functional class, longer duration of AF, and extensive structural remodeling. Those who appear to respond best to catheter ablation have no other structural abnormalities related to their cardiomyopathy. Most of these studies included small numbers of patients and were generally not powered to demonstrate improvements in hard cardiovascular outcomes or all-cause mortality. What is clear from all the trials to date is that HF populations with AF are highly heterogeneous; this can have a significant impact on clinical outcomes. As a result, the major society guidelines have not made specific recommendations about management of these patients with regard to catheter ablation.

Despite significant progress in catheter ablation, a number of unanswered questions remain, including the optimal means of risk stratification of patients with HF to AF ablation, optimal ablation technique in this particular population, and timing of catheter ablation. Whether catheter ablation will be cost-effective in patients with AF and HF remains unclear, especially if patients require multiple re-do procedures, particularly as HF progresses.

Finally, it is important to stress that effective treatment of AF may be achieved only with the simultaneous treatment of heart failure, and vice versa: satisfactory management of AF is essential for the optimum treatment of HF. Thus, it is our well-supported position that using AF ablation first line in patients with HF of any kind is not supported by the literature, clinical experience, or common sense. Given the complexity of both diseases and challenge of conducting studies in the vulnerable patient population, incontrovertible evidence supporting such a position is unlikely to emerge in the foreseeable future.

## REFERENCES

1. Braunwald E. Cardiovascular medicine at the turn of the millennium: triumphs, concerns, and opportunities. N Engl J Med 1997;337:1360–9.
2. National Heart, Lung, and Blood Institute. NHLBI fiscal year 2009 factbook. Bethseda (MD): National Institutes of Health; 2009.
3. American Heart Association Heart Disease, Stroke Statistics Writing Group. Executive summary: heart disease and stroke statistics—2011 update: a report from the American Heart Association. Circulation 2011;123(4):459–63.
4. Benjamin EJ, Levy D, Vaziri SM, et al. Independent risk factors for atrial fibrillation in a population-based cohort: the Framingham Heart Study. JAMA 1994;271(11):840–4.
5. Miyasaka Y, Barnes ME, Gersh BJ, et al. Secular trends in incidence of atrial fibrillation in Olmsted County, Minnesota, 1980 to 2000, and implications on the projections for future prevalence. Circulation 2006;114:119–25.
6. Krijthe BP, Kunst A, Benjamin EJ, et al. Projections on the number of individuals with atrial fibrillation in the European Union, from 2000 to 2060. Eur Heart J 2013;34:2746–51.
7. Chugh SS, Havmoeller R, Narayanan K, et al. Worldwide epidemiology of atrial fibrillation: a Global Burden of Disease 2010 Study. Circulation 2014;129:837–47.
8. Lee Park K, Anter E. Atrial fibrillation and heart failure: a review of the intersection of two cardiac epidemics. J Atr Fibrillation 2013;6(1):751.
9. Carson PE, Johnson GR, Dunkman WB, et al. eFT VA CooperativeStudies Group: The influence of atrial fibrillation on prognosis in mild to moderate heart failure. The V-HeFT Studies. Circulation 1993; 87(Suppl VI):102–10.
10. Middlekauff HR, Stevenson WG, Stevenson LW. Prognostic significance of atrial fibrillation in advanced heart failure. A study of 390 patients. Circulation 1991;84:48–58.
11. Silva-Cardoso J, Zharinov OJ, Ponikowski P, et al, for the RealiseAF Investigators. Heart failure in patients with atrial fibrillation is associated with a high symptom and hospitalization burden: the Realise AF survey. Clin Cardiol 2013;36: 766–74.
12. Lip GY, Laroche C, Popescu MI, et al. Heart failure in patients with atrial fibrillation in Europe: a report from the EUR Observational Research Programme Pilot survey on Atrial Fibrillation. Eur J Heart Fail 2015; 17:570–82.

13. Badheka AO, Rathod A, Kizilbash MA, et al. Comparison of mortality and morbidity in patients with atrial fibrillation and heart failure with preserved versus decreased left ventricular ejection fraction. Am J Cardiol 2011;108:1283–8.

14. Mulder BA, Van Veldhuisen DJ, Crijns HJ, et al, for the RACE II investigators. Lenient vs. strict rate control in patients with atrial fibrillation and heart failure: a post-hoc analysis of the RACE II study. Eur J Heart Fail 2013;15:1311–8.

15. Rahimtoola SH, Ehsani A, Sinno MZ, et al. Left atrial transport function in myocardial infarction. Importance of its booster pump function. Am J Med 1975;59(5):686–94.

16. Raymond RJ, Lee AJ, Messineo FC, et al. Cardiac performance early after cardioversion from atrial fibrillation. Am Heart J 1998;136(3):435–42.

17. Shite J, Yokota Y, Yokoyama M. Heterogeneity and time course of improvement in cardiac function after cardioversion of chronic atrial fibrillation: assessment of serial echocardiographic indices. Br Heart J 1993;70(2):154–9.

18. Pardaens K, Van Cleemput J, Vanhaecke J, et al. Atrial fibrillation is associated with a lower exercise capacity in male chronic heart failure patients. Heart 1997;78:564–8.

19. Clark DM, Plumb VJ, Epstein AE, et al. Hemodynamic effects of an irregular sequence of ventricular cycle lengths during atrial fibrillation. J Am Coll Cardiol 1997;30(4):1039–45.

20. Shinbane JS, Wood MA, Jensen DN, et al. Tachycardia-induced cardiomyopathy: a review of animal models and clinical studies. J Am Coll Cardiol 1997;29(4):709–15.

21. Byrne MJ, Raman JS, Alferness CA, et al. An ovine model of tachycardia-induced degenerative dilated cardiomyopathy and heart failure with prolonged onset. J Card Fail 2002;8(2):108–15.

22. Nerheim P, Birger-Botkin S, Piracha L, et al. Heart failure and sudden death in patients with tachycardia-induced cardiomyopathy and recurrent tachycardia. Circulation 2004;110:247–52.

23. Solti F, Vecsey T, Kékesi V, et al. The effect of atrial dilatation on the genesis of atrial arrhythmias. Cardiovasc Res 1989;23(10):882–6.

24. Eijsbouts SC, Majidi M, van Zandvoort M, et al. Effects of acute atrial dilation on heterogeneity in conduction in the isolated rabbit heart. J Cardiovasc Electrophysiol 2003;14:269–78.

25. Boyden PA, Tilley LP, Albala A, et al. Mechanisms for atrial arrhythmias associated with cardiomyopathy: a study of feline hearts with primary myocardial disease. Circulation 1984;69:1036–47.

26. Ng J, Villuendas R, Cokic I, et al. Autonomic remodeling in the left atrium and pulmonary veins in heart failure—creation of a dynamic substrate for atrial fibrillation. Circ Arrhythm Electrophysiol 2011;4(3):388–96.

27. Li D, Shinagawa K, Pang L, et al. Effects of angiotensin-converting enzyme inhibition on the development of the atrial fibrillation substrate in dogs with ventricular tachypacing–induced congestive heart failure. Circulation 2001;104:2608.

28. Yeh Y, Wakili R, Qi X, et al. Calcium-handling abnormalities underlying atrial arrhythmogenesis and contractile dysfunction in dogs with congestive heart failure. Circ Arrhythm Electrophysiol 2008;1:93–102.

29. Tanaka K, Zlochiver S, Vikstrom KL, et al. Spatial distribution of fibrosis governs fibrillation wave dynamics in the posterior left atrium during heart failure. Circ Res 2007;101:839–47.

30. Sanders P, Morton JB, Davidson NC, et al. Electrical remodeling of the atria in congestive heart failure: electrophysiological and electroanatomic mapping in humans. Circulation 2003;108:1461–8.

31. Li D, Melnyk P, Feng J, et al. Effects of experimental heart failure on atrial cellular and ionic electrophysiology. Circulation 2000;101:2631–8.

32. Cha TJ, Ehrlich JR, Zhang L, et al. Dissociation between ionic remodeling and ability to sustain atrial fibrillation during recovery from experimental congestive heart failure. Circulation 2004;109:412–8.

33. Hsieh MH, Lin YJ, Wang HH, et al. Functional characterization of atrial electrograms in a pacing induced heart failure model of atrial fibrillation: importance of regional atrial connexin40 remodeling. J Cardiovasc Electrophysiol 2013;24:573–82.

34. January CT, Wann LS, Alpert JS, et al. 2014 AHA/ACC/HRS guideline for the management of patients with atrial fibrillation: executive summary: a report of the American College of Cardiology/American Heart Association Task Force on Practice Guidelines and the Heart Rhythm Society. J Am Coll Cardiol 2014;64:2246–80.

35. Pathak RK, Middeldorp ME, Meredith M, et al. Long-term effect of goal-directed weight management in an atrial fibrillation cohort: a long-term follow-up study (LEGACY). J Am Coll Cardiol 2015;65:2159–69.

36. Pathak RK, Middeldorp ME, Lau DH, et al. Aggressive risk factor reduction study for atrial fibrillation and implications for the outcome of ablation: the ARREST-AF cohort study. J Am Coll Cardiol 2014;64:2222–31.

37. Pathak RK, Elliott A, Middeldorp ME, et al. Impact of CARDIOrespiratory FITness on Arrhythmia Recurrence in obese individuals with atrial fibrillation: the CARDIO-FIT Study. J Am Coll Cardiol 2015;66:985–96.

38. Kitzman DW, Brubaker P, Morgan T, et al. Effect of caloric restriction or aerobic exercise training on peak oxygen consumption and quality of life in obese older patients with heart failure with preserved ejection fraction: a randomized clinical trial. JAMA 2016;315:36–46.

39. Kootecha D, Holmes J, Krum H, et al, Beta-Blockers in Heart Failure Collaborative Group. Efficacy of beta blockers in patients with heart failure plus atrial fibrillation: an individual-patient data meta-analysis. Lancet 2014;384:2235–43.

40. Goldberger ZD, Alexander GC. Digitalis use in contemporary clinical practice: refitting the foxglove. JAMA Intern Med 2014;174:151–4.

41. The Digitalis Investigation Group. The effect of digoxin on mortality and morbidity in patients with heart failure. N Engl J Med 1997;336:525–33.

42. Vamos M, Erath JW, Hohnloser SH. Digoxin-associated mortality: a systematic review and meta-analysis of the literature. Eur Heart J 2015. https://doi.org/10.1093/eurheartj/ ehv143.

43. Flory JH, Ky B, Haynes K, et al. Observational cohort study of the safety of digoxin use in women with heart failure. BMJ Open 2012;2:e000888.

44. Gheorghiade M, Fonarow GC, van Veldhuisen DJ, et al. Lack of evidence of increased mortality among patients with atrial fibrillation taking digoxin: findings from post hoc propensity-matched analysis of the AFFIRM trial. Eur Heart J 2013;34:1489–97.

45. Andrey JL, Romero S, García-Egido A, et al. Mortality and morbidity of heart failure treated with digoxin. A propensity-matched study. Int J Clin Pract 2011;65:1250–8.

46. Allen LA, Kowey PR, Piccini JP, et al, ORBIT-AF Investigators. Digoxin use and subsequent outcomes among patients in a contemporary atrial fibrillation cohort. J Am Coll Cardiol 2015;65:2691–8.

47. Echt DS, Liebson PR, Mitchell LB, et al, the CAST Investigators. Mortality and morbidity in patients receiving encainide, flecainide, or placebo: the Cardiac Arrhythmia Suppression Trial. N Engl J Med 1991;324:781–8.

48. Køber L, Torp-Pedersen C, McMurray JJ, et al. Increased mortality after dronedarone therapy for severe heart failure. N Engl J Med 2008;358(25):2678–87.

49. Torp-Pedersen C, Moller M, Bloch-Thomsen PE, et al. Dofetilide in patients with congestive heart failure and left ventricular dysfunction. N Engl J Med 1999;341:857–65.

50. Amiodarone Trials Meta-analysis Investigators: effect of prophylactic amiodarone on mortality after acute myocardial infarction and in congestive heart failure: meta-analysis of individual data from 6500 patients in randomized trials. Lancet 1997;350:1417–24.

51. Pedersen OD, Bagger H, Keller N, et al. Efficacy of dofetilide in the treatment of atrial fibrillation-flutter in patients with reduced left ventricular function. A DIAMOND substudy. Circulation 2001;104:292–6.

52. Deedwania PC, Singh BN, Ellenbogen KA, et al. Spontaneous conversion and maintenance of sinus rhythm by amiodarone in patients with heart failure and atrial fibrillation. Circulation 1998;98:2574–9.

53. Maisel WH, Stevenson LW. Atrial fibrillation in heart failure: epidemiology, pathophysiology, and rationale for therapy. Am J Cardiol 2003;91(6A):2D–8D.

54. Tolosana JM, Hernandez Madrid A, Brugada J, et al. Comparison of benefits and mortality in cardiac resynchronization therapy in patients with atrial fibrillation versus patients in sinus rhythm (Results of the Spanish Atrial Fibrillation and Resynchronization [SPARE] Study). Am J Cardiol 2008;102(4):444–9.

55. Auricchio A, Metra M, Gasparini M, et al. Long-term survival of patients with heart failure and ventricular conduction delay treated with cardiac resynchronization therapy. Am J Cardiol 2007;99(2):232–8.

56. Dickstein K, Bogale N, Priori S, et al. The European cardiac resynchronization therapy survey. Eur Heart J 2009;30(20):2450–60.

57. Carson PE, Johnson GR, Dunkman WB, et al. The influence of atrial fibrillation on prognosis in mild to moderate heart failure. The V-HeFT Studies. The V-HeFT VA Cooperative Studies Group. Circulation 1993;87(6 Suppl):VI102–10.

58. Jędrzejczyk-Patej E, Lenarczyk R, Pruszkowska P, et al. Long-term outcomes of cardiac resynchronization therapy are worse in patients who require atrioventricular junction ablation for atrial fibrillation than in those with sinus rhythm. Cardiol J 2014;21(3):309–15.

59. Healey JS, Hohnloser SH, Exner DV, et al. Cardiac resynchronization therapy in patients with permanent atrial fibrillation: results from the Resynchronization for Ambulatory Heart Failure Trial (RAFT). Circ Heart Fail 2012;5(5):566–70.

60. Gasparini M, Leclercq C, Lunati M, et al. Cardiac resynchronization therapy in patients with atrial fibrillation: the CERTIFY study (cardiac resynchronization therapy in atrial fibrillation patients multinational registry). JACC Heart Fail 2013;1(6):500–7.

61. Brignole M, Pokushalov E, Pentimalli F, et al. A randomized controlled trial of atrioventricular junction ablation and cardiac resynchronization therapy in patients with permanent atrial fibrillation and narrow QRS. Eur Heart J 2018;39(45):3999–4008.

62. Epstein AE, DiMarco JP, Ellenbogen KA, et al. 2012 ACCF/AHA/HRS focused update incorporated into the ACCF/AHA/HRS 2008 guidelines for device-based therapy of cardiac rhythm abnormalities: a report of the American College of Cardiology Foundation/American Heart Association Task Force on Practice Guidelines and the Heart Rhythm Society. J Am Coll Cardiol 2013;61(3):e6–75.

63. Developed with the special contribution of the European Heart Rhythm Association (EHRA), Endorsed by the European Association for Cardio-Thoracic Surgery (EACTS), Authors/Task Force Members,

Camm AJ, Kirchhof P, Lip GY, et al. Guidelines for the management of atrial fibrillation: the Task Force for the Management of Atrial Fibrillation of the European Society of Cardiology (ESC). Eur Heart J 2010; 31(19):2369–429.

64. Calkins H, Hindricks G, Cappato R, et al. 2017 HRS/EHRA/ECAS/APHRS/SOLAECE expert consensus statement on catheter and surgical ablation of atrial. Heart Rhythm 2017;14:10.

65. Liang JJ, Callans DJ. Ablation for atrial fibrillation in heart failure with reduced ejection fraction. Card Fail Rev 2018;4(1):33.

66. Mukherjee RK, Williams SE, Niederer SA, et al. Atrial fibrillation ablation in patients with heart failure: one size does not fit all. Arrhythm Electrophysiol Rev 2018;7(2):84–90.

67. Khan MN, Jaïs P, Cummings J, et al. Pulmonary-vein isolation for atrial fibrillation in patients with heart failure. N Engl J Med 2008;359:1778–85.

68. Di Biase L, Mohanty P, Mohanty S, et al. Ablation versus amiodarone for treatment of persistent atrial fibrillation in patients with congestive heart failure and an implanted device: results from the AATAC multicenter randomized trial. Circulation 2016;133:1637–44.

69. Prabhu S, Taylor AJ, Costello BT, et al. Catheter ablation versus medical rate control in atrial fibrillation and systolic dysfunction: the CAMERA-MRI Study. J Am Coll Cardiol 2017;70:1949–61.

70. Hunter RJ, Berriman TJ, Diab I, et al. A randomized controlled trial of catheter ablation versus medical treatment of atrial fibrillation in heart failure (the CAMTAF trial). Circ Arrhythm Electrophysiol 2014;7:31–8.

71. Marrouche NF, Brachmann J, Andresen D, et al. Catheter ablation for atrial fibrillation with heart failure. N Engl J Med 2018;378(5):417–27.

72. Packer DL, Mark DB, Robb RA, et al. Catheter ablation versus antiarrhythmic drug therapy for atrial fibrillation (CABANA) trial: study rationale and design. Am Heart J 2018;199:192–9.

73. Baher A, Marrouche NF. Treatment of atrial fibrillation in patients with co-existing heart failure and reduced ejection fraction: time to revisit the management guidelines? Arrhythm Electrophysiol Rev 2018;7(2):91.

# Novel Ablation Approaches for Challenging Atrial Fibrillation Cases (Mapping, Irrigation, and Catheters)

Rahul Bhardwaj, MD[a], Jacob S. Koruth, MD[b],*

## KEYWORDS

- Atrial fibrillation ablation • Pulmonary vein isolation • Catheter ablation • Catheter mapping
- Irrigated radiofrequency ablation • Balloon-based catheter ablation • Electroporation

## KEY POINTS

- Catheter ablation technologies for treatment of atrial fibrillation have developed rapidly and along several different lines to fill unmet needs.
- Although in early phases, mapping technologies advances have increased understanding of mechanistic factors in inducing and sustaining atrial fibrillation outside of pulmonary vein triggers and in assessing for gaps in lesion sets.
- New ablation technologies that enable quicker and durable ablation, including single-shot pulmonary vein isolation ablation, also likely will lead to improvements in safety and long-term freedom from atrial fibrillation.

Catheter ablation of atrial fibrillation (AF) has been demonstrated an effective treatment option for symptomatic AF. The most commonly performed procedure within the broad category of AF ablation is pulmonary vein isolation (PVI). Its role in controlling AF has remained central to that of all AF procedures and is essential to AF control because it abolishes the most common source of AF triggers.[1] Although freedom from AF can be achieved with this procedure alone, AF ablation currently remains imperfect with suboptimal success rates.[2] The limitations currently experienced in AF control via ablation stem from shortcomings of current ablation technologies in their ability to create safe and reliably permanent lesions. In addition, in more chronic forms of AF, there exists an incomplete understanding of the mechanisms maintaining AF that can be used to identify specific targets for ablation. This review discusses recent technological advances in AF mapping as well as in catheter ablation.

Broadly, novel approaches to catheter ablation for AF (paroxysmal as well as persistent) can be grouped based on the particular aspect of AF that the technology specifically aims to improve:[1] novel approaches within mapping systems and[2] novel approaches to atrial ablation.

Disclosures: R. Bhardwaj has nothing to disclose. J.S. Koruth is a consultant at Abbott, Farapulse, Vytronus, and Cardiofocus; is on the advisory board at Medtronic and Farapulse; and has research grants from Farapulse, Vytronus, Cardiofocus, and Affera Inc.
a Loma Linda University, 11234 Anderson Street, Room 4404, Loma Linda, CA 92354, USA; b Experimental Lab, Leona M. and Harvey B. Helmsley Electrophysiology Center, Mount Sinai Medical Center, One Gustave L Levy Place - Box 1030, New York, NY 10029, USA
* Corresponding author.
E-mail address: Jacob.koruth@mountsinai.org

0733-8651/19/© 2019 Elsevier Inc. All rights reserved.

cardiology.theclinics.com

## NOVEL APPROACHES WITHIN MAPPING SYSTEMS

Currently used electroanatomic mapping systems include systems that are commonly referred to by the name of their marketed mapping platforms. These include 3 major systems—CARTO (Biosense Webster, Irvine, California), EnSite NavX (St. Jude Medical, St. Paul, Minnesota), and Rhythmia (Boston Scientific, Natick, Massachusetts). Electroanatomic systems use magnetic and impedance information to localize catheters in 3-D space without use of ionizing radiation. Several commercial versions exist within each of these systems and, when looked at broadly, they are primarily designed to provide information on atrial anatomy and tissue voltage. In addition to rendering anatomy in real time, previously acquired CT or MRIs may be integrated into the map, allowing for increased anatomic accuracy, although mapping-based rendering of anatomy has improved to the point that imaging is no longer critical. These maps provide a topographically accurate path for an operator to move the ablation catheter (also visualized within this 3-D map) along the desired areas of the atria. Current systems have automated algorithms that place tags along this path providing not only a road map but also a historical record of all ablations performed. Electroanatomic mapping thus can now be used to assess contiguity of lesions in an accurate manner (**Fig. 1**).

Novel approaches within the systems that either have the potential or have been proven of significant value in improving AF ablation outcomes are briefly highlighted.

## High-density Mapping

The occurrence of recurrent atrial tachycardias (ATs), both focal and macroreentrant, after PVI is not uncommon and is often an unavoidable outcome of ablation strategies used for chronic forms of AF.[3] These ATs can be mapped and successfully eliminated and, therefore, are to long-term arrhythmia-free status of AF ablation patients. High-density mapping refers to the process of mapping of electrical activity through the rapid acquisition of a high number of points that are acquired with catheter with multiple closely spaced electrodes. All major mapping systems offer this feature with system-to-system differences. This technique has transformed the way atypical flutters are approached, in that the automated mapping modules within these systems allow for rapid characterization of complex circuits. High-density maps often helps an operator identify critical sites that sustain the AT, which when ablated often result in durable control of the arrhythmia (**Fig. 2**). Investigators have demonstrated that by using novel ultra–high-density maps, detection of gaps within incomplete PVI lesions sets is improved compared with using traditional high-density maps.[4]

## Atrial Fibrillation Mapping Systems

AF mapping approaches are primarily designed to treat persistent AF, where the role of extra–pulmonary vein (PV) substrate is considered to be significant as PV isolation by itself has been shown to be insufficient for AF control. The systems that are commercially available and those under

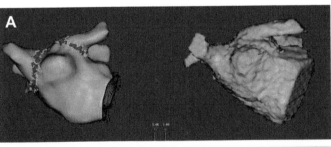
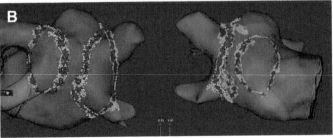

**Fig. 1.** Electroanatomic rendering of left atrial anatomy (*left*) compared with segmented CT scan of the left atrium (*right*) (A). Automated tagging of lesions depicting wide area circumferential PV isolation (B).

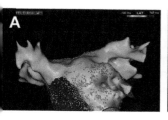
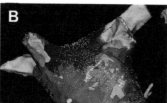

**Fig. 2.** High-density activation map created after PVI demonstrating focal trigger from left atrial appendage after PVI and anterior mitral isthmus ablation (*A*). High-density map of atypical macroreentrant flutter with a multielectrode splined catheter (*B*). The projected points reflect individual activation points acquired in the arrhythmia.

development have been specifically designed to identify sites that are believed critical to maintenance AF. AF mapping systems aim to identify putative drivers of AF, which include focal impulses and reentrant spiral waves (rotors) and thereby offer specific targets for ablation that can improve AF control beyond PVI alone. Spectral analysis is used to localize areas with the highest activation frequencies, which coincide with location of AF foci or rotors. Phase mapping determines the local phase of the activation/recovery cycle at each time point, which enables visualization of spatiotemporally distributed patterns of propagation.[5] The 2 most widely used systems are the focal impulse and rotor modulation system (FIRM) (Abbott, Minneapolis, Minnesota) and the noninvasive panoramic mapping system (CardioInsight, Medtronic, Minneapolis, Minnesota). In addition there are newer mapping systems that use different approaches to AF mapping that are being investigated (**Fig. 3**).

## Focal Impulse and Rotor Modulation System

The FIRM system uses a 64-electrode basket catheter to identify rotational drivers by recording simultaneous intracardiac electrograms in the atrium and uses phase-mapping algorithms to identify focal impulses and rotors. These areas are then ablated with the standard ablation catheter of the operator's choice. Early studies reported widely disparate findings, which has resulted in controversy over its efficacy. The CONFIRM (Conventional Ablation for AF With or Without Focal Impulse and Rotor Modulation) trial included 92 patients with paroxysmal AF or persistent AF and randomized them in a 1:2 fashion to FIRM-guided ablation followed by conventional ablation or conventional ablation alone. The investigators found FIRM-guided ablation had a significantly higher freedom from AF with a single procedure (82.4% vs 44.9%; $P < .001$).[6] At 3 years' follow-up, patients receiving FIRM-guided ablation were found to have high rates of freedom from AF (77.8% vs 38.5%; $P = .001$).[7] In the OASIS (Outcome of Different Ablation Strategies in Persistent and Long-Standing Persistent Atrial Fibrillation) trial, which prospectively evaluating FIRM ablation versus PVI and FIRM versus PVI, posterior wall, and non-PV trigger ablation in nonparoxysmal AF, investigators found that FIRM-guided ablation was inferior at 1 year with regard to freedom from AF (14% vs 52.4% vs 76%, respectively) and that procedures using FIRM were significantly longer.[8] More recently a meta-analysis of 17 studies and 3294 patients using FIRM showed a statistically significant improved odds ratio for freedom from AF with the addition of rotor mapping and ablation. The addition of driver ablation resulted in freedom

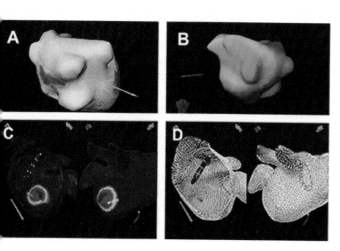

**Fig. 3.** Noninvasive panoramic mapping system driver density (*A*) and phase-array maps (*B*). A rotational driver using an endocardial high-density mapping system is shown (*C, D*).

from AF at 72.5% and from all arrhythmias at 57.8%; when driver ablation was added on to PVI compared with control, the odds ratio of freedom from AF was 3.1 (CI, 1.3–7.7; $P = .02$) and freedom from all arrhythmias of 1.8 (CI, 1.2–2.7; $P<.01$).[9] Due to the conflicting results of studies demonstrating utility of FIRM-based ablation of persistent AF, this approach has not gained widespread acceptance. Additional clinical studies, such as the REAFFIRM and REDO-FIRM clinical trials, are ongoing to provide greater clarity to the effectiveness and clinical utility of this technology.

### Noninvasive Panoramic Mapping

The noninvasive panoramic mapping (CardioInsight, Medtronic) system uses ECGi, a noninvasive technique based on phase analysis of body surface potentials, with a 252-electrode vest worn on the torso combined with noncontrast CT to create high-resolution 3-D patient-specific images of epicardial electrical propagation in AF (see **Fig. 3**). Activation and phase maps are created from unipolar AF electrograms acquired from multiple windows from the vest electrodes during R-R intervals greater than or equal to 1000 ms that are then signal processed to identify drivers. Investigators have reported on 103 consecutive patients with persistent AF who underwent noninvasive mapping to identify drivers. They identified drivers that were ablated in the intervention arm whereas the comparison arm underwent a more traditional ablation approach of stepwise ablation consisting of PVI plus additional ablation. Of the drivers identified, a majority of were reentrant in nature (80.5%), with focal drivers less common (19.5%) Ablation of these drivers terminated AF more commonly in patients with AF of shorter duration. At 12 months, 85% patients with AF termination were free from AF, similar to the control population (87%).[10] In addition, studies have demonstrated that the number of rotors found has been shown associated with the extent of late gadolinium enhancement on cardiac MRI, with clustering near scar borders.[11] Currently this approach is limited by its inability to accurately map septal locations (that remain hidden when viewing the atria from its epicardial aspect) and/or overlapping structures, its spatial accuracy, and its limited resolution for electrograms less than 0.15 mV.[12] Further investigation as well as improving technical aspects are ongoing and its role in persistent AF remains to be established.

### Noninvasive Epicardial and Endocardial Electrophysiology System

A noninvasive epicardial and endocardial electrophysiology system (NEEES) has also been used to identify rotors and focal arrhythmias by creating isopotential and phase maps. This system uses up to 224 unipolar ECG electrodes in special arrays fixed onto a patient's torso, followed by a thoracic MRI performed on the same day. 3-D epicardial and endocardial biatrial geometry is reconstructed with proprietary software (EP Solutions, Yverdon-les-Bains, Switzerland). In a study of 10 patients with persistent AF examining the relationship between rotors detected with noninvasive panoramic mapping and anatomy, rotors based on NEEES analysis were found not regionally associated with areas of late gadolinium enhancement on MRI in contrast to the study done with the CardioInsight system.[13] Further investigation is ongoing at the present time.

Other mapping systems for AF drivers under investigation include a 64-pole basket catheter and offline algorithm to identify reproducible biatrial repetitive activation patterns (CARTOFINDER, Biosense Webster). Early studies have shown this novel technology effective.[14] Another driver mapping technology uses a novel computational high-resolution spatiotemporal mapping algorithm to identify focal impulses and rotors from endocardial signals recorded with a multielectrode catheter in persistent AF (CardioNXT, Westminster, Colorado). By synchronizing multiple sequential samples of electrograms with a conventional mapping catheter, a high-density endocardial contact map is generated. These systems are currently being evaluated and results in terms of AF control remain to be determined.

The field of AF mapping technologies has progressed significantly and continues to grow and evolve. Although some clinical studies performed at select centers have demonstrated utility and efficacy to this approach, these experiences have not been consistently replicated by other investigators and further studies as well as improvements in technical aspects of their mapping approaches are needed to fully understand and address their true potential. Finally, these approaches need to be tested in large multicenter randomized studies to fairly assess their impact on AF outcomes in this challenging population.

## ALTERNATE APPROACHES

Mapping of triggers outside of the PVs has been shown to be effective. Non-PV triggers have been found both in patients with paroxysmal AF and patients with persistent AF.[15] Targeting non-PV triggers after PVI was demonstrated an effective strategy in a prospective study of patients with paroxysmal AF with and without heart failure, with 175 patients in the heart failure arm further divided by PVI alone (n = 87) or PVI and additional non-PV trigger ablation (n = 88). The investigators found long-term freedom from AF at 15.8 months ± 4.7 months superior in the PVI plus non-PV trigger ablation arm (75.0% vs 32.2%; P<.001) and similar to the group of patients without heart failure (75.0% vs 81.7%; P = .44).[16] This study and other studies have brought attention to the concept of adding the search of non-PV triggers as an important step in improving AF control after ablation. Studies of non-PV trigger sources have found the most common sources the left atrial posterior wall, left atrial appendage, ligament of Marshall, superior vena cava, coronary sinus, and crista terminalis. Empiric ablation to isolate these structures is a widely used strategy. The randomized BELIEF trial demonstrated that empiric isolation of the left atrial appendage in long-standing persistent AF can improve long-term freedom from AF and offers another strategy that can help improve AF ablation outcomes in this specific population of AF patients.[17] Isolation of the left atrial appendage remains controversial due to concerns about increased risk of thrombus formation. The aMAZE study to evaluate left atrial appendage ligation using the LARIAT (SentreHEART, Redwood city, CA) device at the time of PVI is ongoing to evaluate efficacy and safety of this technique in persistent AF and long-standing persistent AF.

Several other strategies that do not rely on mapping AF drivers/triggers have been developed to increase the success of catheter ablation of chronic AF beyond PV isolation alone. One approach that has been proposed is a substrate-based ablation targeting areas of scar. The presence of low voltage has been shown to predict recurrence after AF recurrence after ablation in paroxysmal AF (36% vs 6%; hazard ratio 5.89).[18] Investigators have demonstrated that ablation of sites with distinct activation characteristics within/at border zones of LVA in addition to PVI is more effective than conventional PVI-only strategy for persistent AF.[19,20] The ongoing DECAAF II clinical trial is studying conventional PVI versus PVI plus fibrosis-guided ablation, where fibrosis is defined by scar detected by cardiac MRI. Other investigators have proposed using current electro-anatomic mapping systems and multielectrode mapping catheters to identify areas of spatiotemporal dispersion and suggest that targeting these areas for ablation can be an effective strategy for AF termination and, therefore, long-term control.[21] Finally, any discussion of persistent AF ablation strategies would be incomplete without discussing the role of complex fractionated atrial electrograms (CFAEs) ablation. CFAEs can be identified using automated features of these systems as well as by looking for certain ablation catheter characteristics, and early reports suggested this approach to have utility. More recent reports have shown that when added to standard PV ablation, CFAE ablation failed to improve outcomes in paroxysmal AF and persistent AF patients.[22,23] The STAR AF II trial tested PVI alone versus additional CFAE ablation versus additional empiric linear ablation across the left atrial roof and mitral isthmus and found no significant difference in freedom from AF between the 3 strategies at 18 months in patients with persistent AF.[24]

In summary, new mapping approaches and technologies are based on evolving and improved understanding of AF mechanisms. Although some approaches have become more commonplace, some remain confined to limited centers. Although these technologies show promise, further development of each approach as well as further randomized studies are needed to establish their role in AF management. Until then, pursuing PVI in its most complete and durable form remains a reasonable goal.

## NOVEL APPROACHES TO ATRIAL ABLATION

Creation of safe yet consistently transmural atrial ablation lesions is highly desirable not only to achieve durable PVI but also to ensure durable elimination of non-PV targets (triggers and flutter circuits). Reconnection of PVs during redo ablation has been seen in up to 50% of all ablated PVs in early studies.[25] In a systematic review of AF ablation outcomes, the primary mechanism for recurrence found at the time of a repeat procedure was electrical reconnection of the PVs.[26] These findings were supported by the GAP-AF trial, where investigators assigned patients to complete PVI versus incomplete PVI; 117 patients who had complete PVI underwent an invasive reevaluation of the PV 3 months after their index ablation. AF recurred in 62.2% of patients, and, in the 93 patients who underwent the invasive repeat study, 65 (69.9%) of patients were found to have conduction gaps. Among patients who had been randomized to incomplete PVI, the rate of recurrence at 3 months was significantly higher (79.2%) of patients, illustrating the importance and superiority of complete PVI over incomplete isolation.[27] These data reinforce the importance of durable PVI and the need for improvement in existing ablation technology. Modern point-by-point RF ablation and balloon-based ablation techniques are the most commonly used approaches for PV isolation and have yielded improved overall outcomes in recent years due to advances in catheter technology. They do not, however, reliably create permanent transmural lesions in all patients and have other limitations, such as a distal level of isolation with many balloon-based PV isolation technologies. Moreover, these approaches to ablation are not tissue selective for myocardium, in that they also affect adjacent structures, such as the esophagus and phrenic nerve, in pursuit of creating transmural lesions. Several developments have occurred within these established technologies as well as in novel approaches to ablation that have improved the ability to create transmural ablation lesions with reasonable safety (described later).

## Radiofrequency Ablation

Radiofrequency (RF) ablation works by creating resistive heating immediately under the RF catheter tip followed by conductive heating that allows for expansion of the lesion. The size of an ablation lesion is related to the amount of power delivered over time, which in turn is significantly affected by catheter-tissue coupling. Catheter-tissue coupling in turn is determined by the contact force exerted by the catheter tip onto the tissue.[28] Several strategies within the realm of RF ablation have been created to improve outcomes.

### Contact force and radiofrequency indices

Contact force and RF indices refer to the abilities of catheters to provide feedback about contact to tissue and to assess individual ablation points with respect to various parameters, respectively. Clinical studies have demonstrated that ablation with higher contact force correlated with improved clinical outcomes.[29] Contact force–sensing catheters are currently available commercially, and, although these catheters have not been specifically shown to improve outcomes compared with non–force-sensing catheters in large multicenter trials,[30] they have become widely accepted as an essential part of initial AF ablation procedure that involves PV isolation. More importantly, the use of these catheters has allowed for the development of lesion/RF indices that incorporate various parameters essential to lesion formation, such as stability, contact force, impedance drops, and duration of ablation (eg, the force time index). Other scores that are more comprehensive include parameters, such as power (lesion size and ablation index). Together these indices have helped standardize RF delivery, and recent data demonstrate that if ablation is performed using these parameters with strict adherence to lesion proximity, AF outcomes and durable PV isolation rates can be improved.[31] In the PRAISE study, ablation index–guided ablation was performed in 40 consecutive persistent AF patients with a target ablation index of 550 followed by a protocol-mandated repeat procedure in 2 months. PV reconnection was seen in at the repeat electrophysiology study in 22% of patients, affecting 7% of PVs; at 12 months, 95% of patients were in sinus rhythm, with 10% having started antiarrhythmic drugs.[32] The use of this information to track individual ablation points allows operators to manipulate various parameters to reach index targets that correlate to predictable lesions and better outcomes.[33] In conclusion, several studies have demonstrated that the use of force-sensing catheters to create lesions that reach specified targets, and using the contact force information in indices can have a positive impact on the outcome of AF procedures compared with traditional RF delivery approaches with the same/similar catheters.

### Modulation of irrigation in radiofrequency ablation

Irrigation refers to the saline-mediated active cooling of the RF catheter tip that currently is the standard for all ablation catheters used in AF ablation. This is achieved by delivering saline to the tip surface via a variety of designs specific to the catheter tip. Active irrigation mitigates the risk of char formation by actively cooling the catheter tip and thus allowing greater power to be delivered, which in turn improves lesion depth. A risk of this approach, however, is that lesions can be created with excessive depth on the posterior left atrial wall that could result in esophageal injury. Recently, manipulating the flow rate to avoid creating excessively deep lesions on the thin posterior wall of the left atrium has emerged as a strategy to improve safety and avoid esophageal injury. In a recent study, Kumar and colleagues[34] studied lesion characteristics of low-flow ablation in a swine model and evaluated efficacy and safety in a patient cohort. The investigators found that low flow ablation lesions had a greater diameter at the surface compared with high flow, in which greater diameter was found deeper in the tissue. With regard to safety and efficacy, in a clinical comparison between the 166 patients treated with high-flow irrigation and 160 patients treated with low-flow irrigation, there was no difference in acute PVI, complications, or 12-month arrhythmia-free survival between the treatment groups. Titrating flow at the catheter tip to reduce depth on the posterior wall is a feasible and effective option that may reduce risk of esophageal complications.

## High-power, short-duration radiofrequency strategy

The strategy of high-power RF applied for very short durations has recently emerged as an approach to maximize lesion dimensions without excessive depth, capturing an essential requirement for ablation of thin-walled atrial tissue. The rationale for this approach is based on the fact that traditional RF ablation lesions (low–moderate powers for longer durations) are created both by resistive heating immediately under the catheter tip and a zone of conductive heating. A high-power burst of RF, on the other hand, results in a larger resistive heating zone, and the short duration results in shorter temperature decay with reduced conductive heating. This prevents the lesion from acquiring unwanted depth with a corresponding reduction in risk of collateral tissue damage. An ex vivo bovine model used to assess lesion characteristics with either increasing power delivery or duration in the setting of fixed contact force found that although both greater power and longer duration of lesions increased size, the proportional increase in power produced significantly larger lesion volume.[35] In a separate in silico simulation study, high-power, short-duration lesions (50 W/13 s, 60 W/10 s, 70 W/7 s, and 80 W/6 s) were compared with standard RF ablations (30 W/30 s) and similar lesion volumes found. High-power, short-duration lesions, however, had significantly larger diameters and smaller depth.[36] A novel ablation catheter (QDOT MICRO, Biosense Webster) that has multiple thermocouples that allow for catheter tip-tissue temperature measurements has been studied in swine to test a higher-power, short-duration strategy against 25-W/20-second

lesions. High-power ablation (90 W/4 s) resulted in continuous transmural lesions compared with standard catheter ablation that had linear caps in 25% and partial thickness lesions in 29%.[37] Clinically, the high-power, short-duration technique has been validated in a prospective trial of 51 patients with either paroxysmal AF or persistent AF with 50-W ablation lesion achieving lesion size index of 5.5 to 6 and loss of pace capture as a target for ablation endpoint. The study found single-procedure freedom from paroxysmal AF 86% at 2 years and freedom from persistent AF 72% at 2 years.[38] These approaches are currently being prospectively examined. Although this strategy appears attractive in that it can reduce procedure times, its safety and efficacy compared to traditional approaches remains to be convincingly established.

## Temperature-controlled radiofrequency ablation

Newer ablation catheters with unique designs have allowed revisiting temperature-controlled ablation strategies by incorporating temperature sensors, described previously, to detect the temperature at the catheter-tissue interface. This approach to RF delivery uses the temperature data acquired despite the presence of saline irrigation to dynamically alter the power delivered so as to optimize RF delivery. One such catheter (DiamondTemp, Advanced Cardiac Therapeutics, Santa Clara, California) is a composite-tip diamond-embedded irrigated RF catheter with 6 insulated thermocouples on the ablation tip (Fig. 4). The diamond rapidly diffuses heat, and the distal electrode can provide electrograms at higher resolution than standard 3.5-mm or 4-

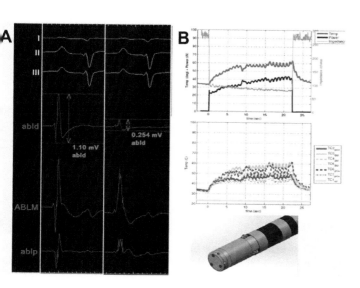

Fig. 4. Temperature-controlled RF ablation demonstrating reduction in catheter tip electrogram (A). Demonstrates the power rising from 25 W to 40 W over the course of this 22-second ablation in a swine experiment (B).

mm ablation catheter electrodes. A preclinical study using this catheter found that ablation performed with a temperature limit of 60°C/50 W resulted in transmurality in 92.7% of atrial lesions. This ablation catheter recently was evaluated in a single-center human feasibility trial for atrial ablation, where RF was delivered in temperature control mode. In this study, 35 patients underwent ablation with the novel catheter and were compared with a cohort of historical patients who had undergone RF ablation using a standard contact force–sensing catheter. PVI was achieved in all patients without any instance of char or thrombus formation. The study cohort had shorter procedures and lower acute dormant PV reconnection rates. At 3 months, at the time of a prespecified remapping procedure done in 23 patients, 84.8% of PV pairs remained durably isolated.[39] This novel technology is currently being evaluated in a multicenter randomized study and further data are needed to understand its true advantages and impact on patient outcomes.

In summary, these and other advances in RF catheter ablation technology have demonstrated improvements in delivery of RF both from safety and efficacy perspectives. This has improved creation of ablation lesions that are tailored to the unique milieu of the atrium. Next-generation ablation catheters that incorporate several of these strategies in a single platform are currently being investigated and offer the prospect of rapid, safe, and durable lesion creation that may have significant impact on procedural workflow, patient safety, and durable outcomes.

### Balloon-based Ablation Catheters

Balloon-based ablation catheters have become a popular alternative to point-by-point RF ablation in that they can achieve PV isolation rapidly and safely with a 1-shot approach and do not require electroanatomic mapping of the chamber. They have been shown safe and noninferior to traditional point-by-point RF ablation in multiple studies. Several balloon catheter technologies are commercially available or are under investigation (**Fig. 5**).

### Cryoballoon

The cryoballoon (Arctic Front Advance Cryoballoon, Medtronic) ablation technique involves occluding PVs individually and decreasing the balloon temperature to freeze tissue and affect tissue necrosis. In the FIRE AND ICE study, cryoballoon ablation was found noninferior to RF ablation in terms of efficacy and had a similar safety profile in a randomized trial of 762 patients with paroxysmal AF; 378 patients were assigned to cryoballoon ablation and 384 patients to the RF ablation arm. At 1.5 years' follow-up, freedom from AF (34.6% vs 35.9%; P<.001 for noninferiority) and safety was similar (10.2% vs 12.8%; P = .24) between both groups.[40] The third-generation cryoballoon (Arctic Front Advance-Short Tip, Medtronic) has been designed with a shorter distal tip (8 mm compared with 13 mm) to facilitate more accurate identification of the time to PVI, which is an

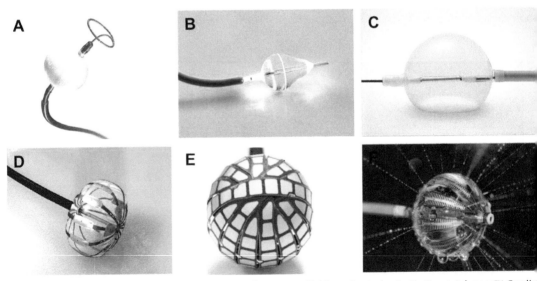

**Fig. 5.** Different balloon catheter ablation systems that are available or in study. Arctic Front Advance™ Cardiac Cryoablation Catheter (A), visually guided laser balloon (B), Satake HotBalloon (C), Apama RF Balloon (D), Kardium Globe (E), and Helios (F) are shown..

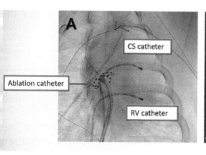 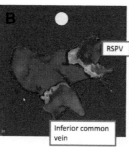

**Fig. 6.** PEF ablation of right superior PV (RSPV) in swine: the fluoroscopic image shows linear pacing catheters in the coronary sinus (CS) and right ventricle (RV) with the PEF ablation catheter in the RSPV (A). The electroanatomic bipolar voltage map shows the RSPV and inferior common vein isolated after ablation: the purple areas demonstrate normal voltage and the red area demonstrates the electrically isolated segments (B).

indicator of acute and durable PVI. A study comparing the second-generation with the third-generation cryoballoon found similar rates of acute PVI but more frequent recorded time to isolation (89.2% vs 60.2%; P<.001), fewer applications (1.6 ± 0.8 vs 1.7 ± 0.8; P = .23), shorter left atrial time (43 min ± 5 min vs 53 min ± 16 min; P<.001), and shorter procedure time (71 min ± 11 min vs 89 min ± 25 min; P<.001).[41] More recently, the cryoballoon has been leveraged for isolating the posterior wall, a frequent target for ablation in persistent AF after PVI. Aryana and colleagues[42] demonstrated the efficacy of this technique in another study of 390 consecutive patients with persistent AF. Posterior wall isolation with cryoballoon was performed and resulted in greater freedom from AF compared with PVI alone. Adjunct RF ablation was necessary to complete posterior wall isolation in 32.4% of patients. Cryoballoon ablation is widely popular and effective, and refinements to catheter technology and new ways of utilizing the balloon technology have expanded its relevance.

## Laser balloon

The visually guided laser balloon (HeartLight, CardioFocus, Marlborough, Massachusetts) is a real-time endoscospic system that similarly involves isolating PVs individually. The balloon is compliant and has variable sizes and is inflated with fluid. The balloon is used to occlude the target PV, and 980-nm laser energy is delivered with a maneuverable 30° light arc to ablate tissue. It has been validated in clinical studies for paroxysmal AF[43] and persistent AF,[44] with efficacy similar to conventional RF ablation. The pivotal multicenter clinical trial randomized 353 patients to ablation with the visually guided laser balloon or conventional RF ablation. The primary efficacy endpoint, which included freedom from recurrent arrhythmia, failure to isolate all PVs, and use of antiarrhythmic drugs, was met in 61.1% of the balloon arm versus 61.7% in controls (P = .003), and the safety endpoint was met, although diaphragmatic paralysis was significantly higher in the laser balloon

arm.[45] Long-term outcomes after laser balloon ablation also have been reported. In a cohort of 90 patients, 5-year freedom rates from arrhythmia recurrence after a single procedure was 51% and 78% respectively with multiple procedures.[46] A multicenter remapping study to assess durability of PVI with the laser balloon was performed in 52 patients after 105 days ± 44 days and found 162 of 189 (86%) PVs remained isolated and 32 of 52 (62%) of patients had all PVs isolated. The likelihood of achieving durable PVI differed among operators who performed fewer than 10 procedures versus those who performed more than 10 (73% vs 89%; P = .011).[47] Laser balloon has demonstrated effective for PVI and, more recently, a third generation laser balloon (HeartLight X3, CardioFocus) has been developed that can create rapid, uninterrupted and continuous lesions and is being currently investigated. Although limited by tissue selectivity, the laser balloon represents an alternative solution to achieving rapid PVI.

## HotBalloon

The hot balloon ablation system (SATAKE HotBalloon, Toray Industries, Tokyo, Japan) uses thermal energy from a heated compliant balloon to ablate tissue. The balloon is heated with RF energy generated from a coil electrode on the catheter shaft that agitates fluid inside the balloon. In a prospective randomized controlled study of 143 patients with paroxysmal AF, 100 were randomized to the hot balloon and 43 were randomized to antiarrhythmic drug therapy. Acute PVI was achieved in 98% of veins in 93% of patients in the hot balloon arm. At 9 months' follow-up, chronic success defined as freedom from AF was demonstrated in 59.0% of the hot balloon arm compared with 4.7% of the antiarrhythmic therapy arm. In terms of safety, the rate of major complications was 11.2%, including PV stenosis (5.2%) and phrenic nerve injury (3.7%).[48] Subsequent clinical trials have similar efficacy results, although often additional touch-up RF lesions were needed for complete PV isolation.[49]

### Novel radiofrequency balloons

Several novel irrigated balloon-based catheters that deploy RF energy are currently undergoing clinical investigation and appear promising. One such balloon, is an endoscopic balloon catheter system (Apama Radiofrequency Balloon Catheter System, Boston Scientific) that has multipoint RF delivery capabilities that facilitate single-shot PVI as well as potentially linear or focal ablation. Early data from a first-in-man trial, AF-FICIENT, has suggested both safety and efficacy with short procedural times. Another novel irrigated RF balloon catheter (Helios, Biosense Webster) allows for directionally tailored energy delivery for PVI by customizing the amount of energy delivered at chosen locations in an attempt to reduce the risk of collateral injury. Early safety and efficacy for this catheter for PVI was demonstrated in the multicenter RADIANCE feasibility study. Finally, a multielectrode array catheter (Globe Mapping and Ablation System, Kardium, Burnaby, British Columbia, Canada) that has 122 flat electrodes on an expanding, contact-based, semicompliant array has also been developed. This system can create high density activation and voltage maps, is able to pace as well as deploy RF to ablate tissue. An early feasibility study demonstrated efficacy and safety and further studies are ongoing.

## Alternative Energy Sources

### Irreversible electroporation or pulse electric field ablation

The novel and investigational energy source, irreversible electroporation, or pulse electric field (PEF) ablation, ablates tissue via a nonthermal mechanism, that is, by creating permanent microscopic pores in cell membranes that result in cell death. This energy source has been used to ablate tumors and has recently been investigated in preclinical models for cardiac ablation. PEF is unique in that it spares the extracellular matrix and has tissue-specific effects, a combination that allows for ablation of targeted myocardium only, with a very low risk for collateral injury, as indicated by preclinical experience so far. There are significant preclinical data supporting the safety of irreversible electroporation/PEF in the context of the esophagus, phrenic nerve, coronary arteries, and PV stenosis[50–54] (Fig. 6). Recently, first-in-human studies have been undertaken that have demonstrated that PEF-based PV ablation is feasible and safe. This early work was a small single-center study that reported only acute procedural outcomes.[55] Significant work needs to be done in this field

and its ultimate role as an ablation therapy remains to be further defined.

## The Role of Esophageal Protection

Esophageal injury is an uncommon but potentially life-threatening adverse event associated with AF ablation due to the close proximity of the posterior left atrium to the esophagus. The authors strongly believe this is an important area that needs to be considered in the realm of novel ablation technologies that use thermal ablative mechanism. The high mortality rates associated with a particularly extreme form of esophageal injury, the atrioesophageal fistula, should serve as an important reminder of the severe consequences of esophageal injury, and this risk should be constantly and carefully evaluated as new ablation technologies evolve. An atrioesophageal fistula occurs when esophageal tissue is thermally injured and necrosis occurs, eventually ulcerating and forming a connection between the esophageal lumen and left atrium.[56] One of the more common strategies used for esophageal protection is that of monitoring luminal esophageal temperatures during ablation. Several probes are available for this purpose, including single-thermistor and multithermistor probes. The advantage of multithermistor probes with greater sensitivity is earlier detection of temperature elevation. More recently, several strategies of esophageal deviation to prevent injury have been described.[57,58] These novel technologies prevent esophageal injury by moving the esophagus physically away from the area of ablation.

## SUMMARY

Catheter ablation technologies for treatment of AF have developed rapidly and along several different lines to fill unmet needs. New ablation technologies including single-shot PVI approaches are designed to enable quicker and durable ablation lesions and will likely lead to improvements in long-term freedom from AF. This as well as their safety remains to be established at this time. Although early results are encouraging, clinical trials are needed to validate these new tools.

## REFERENCES

1. Haïssaguerre M, Jaïs P, Shah DC, et al. Spontaneous initiation of atrial fibrillation by ectopic beat originating in the pulmonary veins. N Engl J Med 1998;339:659–66.
2. Pallisgaard JL, Gislason GH, Hansen J, et al. Temporal trends in atrial fibrillation recurrence rates after

ablation between 2005 and 2014: a nationwide Danish cohort study. Eur Heart J 2018;39(6):442–9.

3. Wasmer K, Mönnig G, Bittner A, et al. Incidence, characteristics, and outcome of left atrial tachycardias after circumferential antral ablation of atrial fibrillation. Heart Rhythm 2012;9:1660–6.

4. Anter E, Tschabrunn CM, Contreras-Valdes FM, et al. Pulmonary vein isolation using the Rhythmia mapping system: verification of intracardiac signals using the Orion mini-basket catheter. Heart Rhythm 2015;12(9):1927–34.

5. Quintanilla JG, Pérez-Villacastín J, Pérez-Castellano N, et al. Mechanistic approaches to detect, target, and ablate the drivers of atrial fibrillation. Circ Arrhythm Electrophysiol 2016;9(1):e002481.

6. Narayan SM, Krummen DE, Shivkumar K, et al. Treatment of atrial fibrillation by the ablation of localized sources: CONFIRM (conventional ablation for atrial fibrillation with or without focal impulse and rotor modulation) trial. J Am Coll Cardiol 2012; 60(7):628–36.

7. Narayan SM, Baykaner T, Clopton P, et al. Ablation of rotor and focal sources reduces late recurrence of atrial fibrillation compared with trigger ablation alone: extended follow-up of the CONFIRM trial (conventional ablation for atrial fibrillation with or without focal impulse and rotor modulation). J Am Coll Cardiol 2014;63(17):1761–8.

8. Mohanty S, Gianni C, Mohanty P, et al. Impact of rotor ablation in nonparoxysmal atrial fibrillation patients results from the randomized OASIS trial. J Am Coll Cardiol 2016;68:274–82 (RETRACTED).

9. Baykenar T, Rogers AJ, Meckler GL, et al. Clinical implications of ablation of drivers for atrial fibrillation: a systematic review and meta-analysis. Circ Arrhythm Electrophysiol 2018;11(5):1–10.

10. Haissaguerre M, Hocini M, Denis A, et al. Driver domains in persistent atrial fibrillation. Circulation 2014; 130(7):530–8.

11. Cochet H, Dubois R, Yamashita S, et al. Relationship between fibrosis detected on late gadolinium-enhanced cardiac magnetic resonance and re-entrant activity assessed with electrocardiographic imaging in human persistent atrial fibrillation. JACC Clin Electrophysiol 2018;4(1):17–29.

12. Lim HS, et al. The utility of noninvasive mapping in persistent atrial fibrillation ablation. In: Practical guide to catheter ablation of atrial fibrillation. 2nd edition. Wiley Blackwell; 2015.

13. Sohns C, Lemes C, Metzner A, et al. First-in-man analysis of the relationship between electrical rotors from noninvasive panoramic mapping and atrial fibrosis from magnetic resonance imaging in patients with persistent atrial fibrillation. Circ Arrhythm Electrophysiol 2017;10(8):e004419.

14. Honarbakhsh S, Schilling RJ, Dhillon G, et al. A novel mapping system for panoramic mapping of the left atrium application to detect and characterize localized sources maintaining atrial fibrillation. JACC Clin Electrophysiol 2018;4(1): 124–34.

15. Santangeli P, Zado ES, Hutchinson MD, et al. Prevalence and distribution of focal triggers in persistent and long-standing persistent atrial fibrillation. Heart Rhythm 2016;13(2):374–82.

16. Zhao Y, Di Biase L, Trivedi C, et al. Importance of non–pulmonary vein triggers ablation to achieve long-term freedom from paroxysmal atrial fibrillation in patients with low ejection fraction. Heart Rhythm 2016;13(1):141–9.

17. Di Biase L, Burkhardt JD, Mohanty P, et al. Left atrial appendage isolation in patients with longstanding persistent af undergoing catheter ablation: BELIEF trial. J Am Coll Cardiol 2016;68(18):1929–40.

18. Masuda M, Fujita M, Iida O, et al. Left atrial low-voltage areas predict atrial fibrillation recurrence after catheter ablation in patients with paroxysmal atrial fibrillation. Int J Cardiol 2018;257: 97–101.

19. Rolf S, Kircher S, Arya A, et al. Tailored atrial substrate modification based on low-voltage areas in catheter ablation of atrial fibrillation. Circ Arrhythm Electrophysiol 2014;7(5):825–33.

20. Jadidi AS, Lehrmann H, Keyl C, et al. Ablation of persistent atrial fibrillation targeting low-voltage areas with selective activation characteristics. Circ Arrhythm Electrophysiol 2016;9(3):e002962.

21. Seitz J, Bars C, Théodore G, et al. AF ablation guided by spatiotemporal electrogram dispersion without pulmonary vein isolation: a wholly patient-tailored approach. J Am Coll Cardiol 2017;69(3): 303–21.

22. Bassiouni M, Saliba W, Hussein A, et al. Randomized study of persistent atrial fibrillation ablation: ablate in sinus rhythm versus ablate complex-fractionated atrial electrograms in atrial fibrillation. Circ Arrhythm Electrophysiol 2016;9(2):e003596.

23. Providencia R, Lambiase PD, Srinivasan N, et al. Is there still a role for complex fractionated atrial electrogram ablation in addition to pulmonary vein isolation in patients with paroxysmal and persistent atrial fibrillation? meta-analysis of 1415 patients. Circ Arrhythm Electrophysiol 2015;8(5):1017–29.

24. Verma A, Jiang CY, Betts TR, et al. Approaches to catheter ablation for persistent atrial fibrillation. N Engl J Med 2015;372:1812–22.

25. Cheema A, Dong J, Dalal D, et al. Incidence and time course of early recovery of pulmonary vein conduction after catheter ablation of atrial fibrillation. J Cardiovasc Electrophysiol 2007;18(4):387–91.

26. Ganesan AN, Shipp NJ, Brooks AG, et al. Long-term outcomes of catheter ablation of atrial fibrillation: a systemic review and meta-analysis. J Am Heart Assoc 2013;2:e004549.

27. Kuck KH, Hoffmann BA, Ernst S, et al. Impact of complete versus incomplete circumferential lines around the pulmonary veins during catheter ablation of paroxysmal atrial fibrillation: results from the gap-atrial fibrillation–German atrial fibrillation competence network 1 trial. Circ Arrhythm Electrophysiol 2016;9(1):e003337.

28. Yokoyama K, Nakagawa H, Shah DC, et al. Novel contact force sensor incorporated in irrigated radiofrequency ablation catheter predicts lesion size and incidence of steam pop and thrombus. Circ Arrhythm Electrophysiol 2008;1(5):354–62.

29. Reddy VY, Shah D, Kautzner J, et al. The relationship between contact force and clinical outcome during radiofrequency catheter ablation of atrial fibrillation in the TOCCATA study. Heart Rhythm 2012;9(11): 1789–95.

30. Reddy VY, Dukkipati SR, Neuzil P, et al. Randomized, controlled trial of the safety and effectiveness of a contact force-sensing irrigated catheter for ablation of paroxysmal atrial fibrillation: results of the TactiCath Contact Force Ablation Catheter Study for Atrial Fibrillation (TOCCASTAR) study. Circulation 2015;132:907–15.

31. Mattia L, Crosato M, Indiani S, et al. Prospective evaluation of lesion index-guided pulmonary vein isolation technique in patients with paroxysmal atrial fibrillation: 1-year follow-up. J Atr Fibrillation 2018; 10(6):1858.

32. Hussein A, Das M, Riva S, et al. Use of ablation index-guided ablation results in high rates of durable pulmonary vein isolation and freedom from arrhythmia in persistent atrial fibrillation patients: the praise study results. Circ Arrhythm Electrophysiol 2018;11(9):e006576.

33. Taghji P, El Haddad M, Phlips T, et al. Evaluation of a strategy aiming to enclose the pulmonary veins with contiguous and optimized radiofrequency lesions in paroxysmal atrial fibrillation: a pilot study. JACC Clin Electrophysiol 2018;4(1):99–108.

34. Kumar S, Romero J, Stevenson WG, et al. Impact of lowering irrigation flow rate on atrial lesion formation in thin atrial tissue: preliminary observations from experimental and clinical studies. JACC Clin Electrophysiol 2017;3(10):1115–25.

35. Borne RT, Sauer WH, Zipse MM, et al. Longer duration versus increasing power during radiofrequency ablation yields different ablation lesion characteristics. JACC Clin Electrophysiol 2018;4(7):902–8.

36. Bourier F, Duchateau J, Vlachos K, et al. High-power short-duration versus standard radiofrequency ablation: insights on lesion metrics. J Cardiovasc Electrophysiol 2018. https://doi.org/10.1111/jce.13724.

37. Leshem E, Zilberman I, Tschabrunn CM, et al. High-power and short-duration ablation for pulmonary vein isolation: biophysical characterization. JACC Clin Electrophysiol 2018;4(4):467–79.

38. Winkle RA, Moskovitz R, Hardwin Mead R, et al. Atrial fibrillation ablation using very short duration 50 W ablations and contact force sensing catheters. J Interv Card Electrophysiol 2018;52(1):1–8.

39. Iwasawa J, Koruth JS, Petru J, et al. Temperature-controlled radiofrequency ablation for pulmonary vein isolation in patients with atrial fibrillation. J Am Coll Cardiol 2017;70(5):542–53.

40. Kuck KH, Brugada J, Fürnkranz A, et al. Cryoballoon or radiofrequency ablation for paroxysmal atrial fibrillation. N Engl J Med 2016;374:2235–45.

41. Aryana A, Kowalski M, O'Neill PG, et al. Catheter ablation using the third-generation cryoballoon provides an enhanced ability to assess time to pulmonary vein isolation facilitating the ablation strategy: short- and long-term results of a multicenter study. Heart Rhythm 2016;13(12):2306–13.

42. Aryana A, Baker JH, Espinosa Ginic MA, et al. Posterior wall isolation using the cryoballoon in conjunction with pulmonary vein ablation is superior to pulmonary vein isolation alone in patients with persistent atrial fibrillation: a multicenter experience. Heart Rhythm 2018;15(8):1121–9.

43. Dukkipati SR, Kuck KH, Neuzil P, et al. Pulmonary vein isolation using a visually guided laser balloon catheter the first 200-patient multicenter clinical experience. Circ Arrhythm Electrophysiol 2013; 6(3):467–72.

44. Schmidt B, Neuzil P, Luik A, et al. Laser balloon or wide-area circumferential irrigated radiofrequency ablation for persistent atrial fibrillation: a multicenter prospective randomized study. Circ Arrhythm Electrophysiol 2017;10(12):1–10.

45. Dukkipati SR, Cuoco F, Kutinsky I, et al. Pulmonary vein isolation using the visually guided laser balloon a prospective, multicenter, and randomized comparison to standard radiofrequency ablation. J Am Coll Cardiol 2015;66(12):1350–60.

46. Reissmann B, Budelmann T, Wissner E, et al. Five year clinical outcomes of visually guided laser balloon pulmonary vein isolation for the treatment of paroxysmal atrial fibrillation. Clin Res Cardiol 2018;107(5):405–12.

47. Dukkipati SR, Neuzil P, Kautzner J, et al. The durability of pulmonary vein isolation using the visually guided laser balloon catheter: multicenter results of pulmonary vein remapping studies. Heart Rhythm 2012;9:919–25.

48. Sohara H, Ohe T, Okumura K, et al. HotBalloon ablation of the pulmonary veins for paroxysmal AF: multicenter randomized trial in Japan. J Am Coll Cardiol 2016;68(25):2747–57.

49. Sohara H, Takeda H, Ueno H, et al. Feasibility of the radiofrequency hot balloon catheter for isolation of the posterior left atrium and pulmonary veins for the treatment of atrial fibrillation. Circ Arrhythm Electrophysiol 2009;2:225–32.

50. Wittkampf FH, van Driel VJ, van Wessel H, et al. Feasibility of electroporation for the creation of pulmonary vein ostial lesions. J Cardiovasc Electrophysiol 2011;22:302–9.

51. van Driel VJ, Neven KG, van Wessel H, et al. Pulmonary vein stenosis after catheter ablation: electroporation versus radiofrequency. Circ Arrhythm Electrophysiol 2014;7:734–8.

52. Neven K, van Driel V, van Wessel H, et al. Safety and feasibility of closed chest epicardial catheter ablation using electroporation. Circ Arrhythm Electrophysiol 2014;7:913–9.

53. du Pré BC, van Driel VJ, van Wessel H, et al. Minimal coronary artery damage by myocardial electroporation ablation. Europace 2012;15:144–9.

54. Neven K, van Es R, van Driel V, et al. Acute and long-term effects of full-power electroporation ablation directly on the porcine esophagus. Circ Arrhythm Electrophysiol 2017;10:e004672.

55. Reddy VY, Koruth J, Jais P, et al. Ablation of atrial fibrillation with pulsed electric fields: an ultra-rapid, tissue-selective modality for cardiac ablation. JACC Clin Electrophysiol 2018;4(8):987–95.

56. Chavez P, Messerli FH, Casso Dominguez A, et al. Atrioesophageal fistula following ablation procedures for atrial fibrillation: systematic review of case reports. Open Heart 2015;2:e000257.

57. Bhardwaj R, Naniwadekar A, Whang W, et al. Esophageal deviation during atrial fibrillation ablation: clinical experience with a dedicated esophageal balloon retractor. JACC Clin Electrophysiol 2018; 4(8):1020–30.

58. Parikh V, Swarup V, Hantla J, et al. Feasibility, safety, and efficacy of a novel preshaped nitinol esophageal deviator to successfully deflect the esophagus and ablate left atrium without esophageal temperature rise during atrial fibrillation ablation: the DEFLECT GUT study. Heart Rhythm 2018;15(9):1321–7.

# Prediction and Management of Recurrences after Catheter Ablation in Atrial Fibrillation and Heart Failure

Majd A. El-Harasis, MBBS[a],
Christopher V. DeSimone, MD, PhD[b], Xiaoxi Yao, PhD[c,d],
Peter A. Noseworthy, MD[b,d],*

## KEYWORDS

• Heart failure • Catheter ablation • Atrial fibrillation • Cardiac resynchronization therapy

## KEY POINTS

• Atrial fibrillation (AF) ablation is an effective method of rhythm control, but heart failure patients are particularly prone to have recurrence post-ablation.
• Individual patient characteristics that may be used to determine risk of recurrence include left atrial volume and scarring, ECG parameters, timing of recurrence, and serum biomarkers.
• The role of cardiac MRI in predicting the risk of recurrence is being increasingly recognized because it can aid in determining the degree of left atrial scarring, volume, and sphericity.
• Management of AF recurrence can also be achieved by pharmacologic therapy and through AV nodal ablation with pacing.

## CATHETER ABLATION OF ATRIAL FIBRILLATION IN PATIENTS WITH HEART FAILURE

### Introduction

As the prevalence of atrial fibrillation (AF) and heart failure (HF) continues to rise, patients with coexistence of these conditions are increasingly common. In patients with HF, concomitant AF portends a higher mortality, with a 9.5-fold increase in mortality within the first 4 months of AF diagnosis.[1] Currently, catheter ablation is recommended in patients with symptomatic AF refractory to antiarrhythmic drugs (AADs), an approach that is being used increasingly given the suboptimal efficacy of AADs, which is around 65% effective at 3 years.[2,3]

Multiple studies, including randomized clinical trials and meta-analyses, have demonstrated the efficacy of catheter ablation in patients with coexistent HF and AF.[4–10] More recently, a randomized clinical trial by Marrouche and colleagues[11] (CASTLE-AF) examined catheter ablation versus medical management in 363 patients with New York Heart Association (NYHA) functional class

Disclosure Statement: None of the authors have any disclosures.
[a] Division of Internal Medicine, Mayo Clinic, 200 First Street Southwest, Rochester, MN 55905, USA; [b] Department of Cardiovascular Diseases, Mayo Clinic, 200 First Street Southwest, Rochester, MN 55905, USA; [c] Division of Health Care Policy and Research, Department of Health Sciences Research, Mayo Clinic, 200 First Street Southwest, Rochester, MN 55905, USA; [d] Robert D. and Patricia E. Kern Center for the Science of Health Care Delivery, Mayo Clinic, 200 First Street Southwest, Rochester, MN 55905, USA
* Corresponding author. Division of Cardiovascular Diseases, Mayo Clinic College of Medicine, 200 First Street Southwest, Rochester, MN 55905.
E-mail address: noseworthy.peter@mayo.edu

II-IV HF with an ejection fraction (EF) less than or equal to 35% and demonstrated a reduction in the composite end point of all-cause mortality or hospitalization for worsening HF (28.5% vs 44.6%; hazard ratio, 0.62; 95% confidence interval [CI], 0.43–0.87; $P = .007$) in the ablation group. When examined separately, there was a significant reduction in each of the outcomes of all-cause mortality, HF hospitalizations, and cardiovascular mortality. The CABANA trial, which has randomized more than 2200 patients with AF, of which approximately 15% had HF, to catheter ablation versus pharmacologic rhythm control, has not yet been published but will likely add considerably to the understanding of the role for ablation in this population.[12]

Given the propensity for AF to recur post-ablation, the importance of understanding patient factors that increase the risk for recurrence and/or ablation failure has been increasingly apparent. This review delineates predictors of AF recurrence in patients with HF and subsequent management of patients with recurrence.

### Challenges in Atrial Fibrillation Ablation in Patients with Heart Failure

AF recurrence remains a difficult, but common clinical scenario in patients with HF. Prior reports note that 20% to 40% of patients, including those without a history of congestive heart failure, who undergo ablation require a repeat procedure.[13,14] Wilton and colleagues[7] performed a meta-analysis on AF catheter ablation in patients with left ventricular (LV) systolic dysfunction, as compared with those without. This included eight studies (1851 patients) and demonstrated that patients with and without HF with reduced EF (HFrEF) had a similar risk for recurrence of AF but more procedures were required in HFrEF patients. The relative risk for recurrence in those with and without HFrEF was 1.5 (95% CI, 1.2–1.8) after one procedure and 1.2 (95% CI, 0.9–1.5) after multiple procedures. Importantly, there was no difference in complications ($P = .55$). In addition, they found a pooled absolute improvement of 11% in LVEF in patients with HFrEF (95% CI, 7%–14%; $P<.001$) with ablation. It should be noted, that seven out of eight studies included in this meta-analysis came from single-center observational studies with high volumes of catheter ablations, raising the question of whether the inclusion of less experienced centers would have altered the results, and if these findings could be extrapolated to less experienced or lower volume centers.

HF results in structural and functional changes that can alter the success rate of ablation.

Currently, AF ablation is typically performed via circumferential ablative lesions within the left atrial (LA) myocardium just outside the pulmonary veins (PV), so-called "antral" ablation, with the goal of isolation of vein from LA tissue.[15] However, in patients with HF, progressive changes in the left atrium result in additional regions of the atrium, in addition to the PVs, that can trigger AF.[16] These changes include volume and pressure overload, resulting in atrial stretch and progressive interstitial fibrosis. In addition, impairment of LA function results in changes in structural proteins within the myocytes, and changes in ion channel composition that occur during the remodeling process.[17] The latter results in triggered activity and delayed afterdepolarizations, which is thought to be one mechanism by which AF is initiated in these patients.[18] An additional factor is the progression of paroxysmal AF to persistent AF in a substantial number of patients, perhaps because of progressive atrial fibrosis, a process that HF has been shown to accelerate.[19]

Additional adjunctive ablation strategies include linear ablation (similar to the surgical Cox maze procedure), complex fractionated atrial electrogram based ablation, rotor ablation, scar-based ablation and ablation of non-PV triggers, commonly located in the coronary sinus, LA appendage, right atrium and superior vena cava.[20–24] However, previous studies in patients without HF have shown mixed results with some showing no additional benefit with empiric linear ablation or complex fractionated atrial electrogram-based ablation,[25] but their exact benefit and utility in patients with HFrEF remains to be determined.

The autonomic system, which is altered in patients with HF, has also been suggested to play a role. In HF, there is activation of the sympathetic nervous system and reduction in vagal activity, resulting in an upregulation of the renin angiotensin-aldosterone system.[26] The association between abnormal autonomic innervation and AF has been demonstrated in animal and human models. One study in dogs demonstrated increased sympathetic nerve densities in dogs with sustained AF.[27] There has also been shown to be increased sympathetic nerve densities in humans with chronic AF, based on histopathologic studies.[28]

Modulation of the autonomic nervous system has been studied in models of AF. Ablation of the left and right stellate ganglia along with the superior cardiac branch of the left thoracic vagal nerve in a canine model resulted in a delay (but not prevention) in the development of AF after atrial tachy-pacing.[29] However, there are weaknesses to this model that limit the direct translation of these findings to humans. Notably, these models do not take into account additional AF risk factors, such as hypertension, HF, and obesity, that would prevail in humans, and fails to account for the fact that these sympathetic ganglia are not easy to access in humans.[30]

## PREDICTORS OF ATRIAL FIBRILLATION RECURRENCE IN PATIENTS WITH HEART FAILURE

AF and HF share key underlying pathophysiologic drivers including myocardial hypertrophy, fibrosis and apoptosis, neurohormonal activation, and elevated filling pressures, in addition to common risk factors, such as obesity, hypertension, and ischemic heart disease,[31] thereby exhibiting a bidirectional pathophysiologic relationship. Furthermore, tachycardia-induced cardiomyopathy and loss of atrioventricular (AV) synchrony with subsequent suboptimal ventricular filling can further potentiate HF.[31] Of note, there does not seem to be a difference in arrhythmia-free recurrence or functional improvement between patients with HF with reduced EF compared with preserved EF.[32] The exact degree by which each condition drives the other is unknown, but given the propensity for AF to recur following ablation, there has been increasing interest in defining individual patient characteristics that may portend a higher risk of recurrence.

### Left Atrial Volume and Scarring

LA volume has been shown to correlate with risk of AF recurrence. A meta-analysis performed by Njoku and colleagues[33] demonstrated that patients who developed recurrence of their AF had a higher LA volume (11 studies with 1559 patients) and LA volume index (nine studies with 1425 subjects). Furthermore, a meta-analysis performed by Zhuang and colleagues[34] showed that there were significantly lower LA volumes and diameters postablation without significant differences in LA EF and strain preablation and postablation. These significantly lower volumes persisted in patients without AF recurrence but not in patients who experienced a recurrence. However, given the inconsistencies in the data, there is no definitive LA size cutoff beyond which one can clearly say that ablation would not be worth pursuing.[16]

The structural and functional remodeling of the LA seems much more complex than what is ascribed to simple volumetric assessments. Scar tissue within the LA has been postulated as a key driver of AF recurrence. It has been shown that atrial fibrosis and scarring in HF alters atrial conduction and the duration of the effective refractory period,[35] which has been shown to strongly promote progression toward more sustained AF.[36] In addition, scarring may render the atrial tissue more vulnerable to AF induction by sources other than the tissue surrounding the PVs,[37] which may be related to differences in coupling intervals and timing of ectopic beats.[38] Furthermore, fibrotic atria are more likely to develop AF by burst or premature atrial pacing compared with normal hearts.[39]

The ideal ablation-related scar volume and location that would prevent AF recurrence without reducing LA function is unknown.[34] Peters and colleagues[40] have shown that patients with more scarring in the area of the right inferior PV had less recurrence of AF. However, Wylie and coworkers[41] showed that overall more scar correlated with reduced LA function. Verma and coworkers[37] has shown that patients with LA scarring (covering an average of 21 ± 11% of the LA surface) was the only independent predictor of AF recurrence, by multivariate analysis. Ablation-related atrial injury can result in reductions in atrial function and compliance, which can increase pulmonary venous pressures and result in dyspnea, a phenomenon termed "stiff left atrium syndrome."[42] Further research is required to optimize knowledge of the ideal scar burden and location.

### Arrhythmia Termination During the Index Ablation Procedure

Procedural termination of AF has been shown to herald lower rates of recurrence.[43] This also held true in patients with persistent AF, because Park and colleagues[44] demonstrated that patients with persistent AF who had AF terminated during their index procedure had a lower recurrence rate over a follow-up period of 18.7 ± 7.6 months compared with those in whom AF did not terminate (45.3% vs 68.9%; $P = .009$). Of note, in the previously mentioned study by Verma and coworkers,[37] in a subgroup analysis, scarring was not shown to be associated with an inability to achieve the end point of PV isolation.

### Electrocardiogram Parameters

Ma and colleagues[45] studied P wave duration, P wave dispersion (difference between the maximum and minimum P wave duration among all measurable electrocardiogram leads), and the interval from electrocardiogram P wave onset to LA appendage ejection flow determined by echocardiography in 136 patients with AF who converted to sinus rhythm either spontaneously or following electrical cardioversion. These parameters were significantly longer in patients who developed recurrence during their follow-up period of 12 ± 6 months. Other factors that have been studied in the setting of recurrence following cardioversion include fibrillation frequency, because patients with lower fibrillatory frequency were more likely to convert to sinus rhythm spontaneously, respond to drug therapy, and remain in sinus rhythm following cardioversion.[46,47] In addition, dispersion of AF cycle lengths was noted to be significantly higher in those with recurrence.[48]

### Early Recurrence

Cai and colleagues[49] demonstrated that patients with early AF recurrence (which was defined as within 3 months of ablation) was an independent predictor of later recurrence. Similarly, Bertaglia and colleagues[50] demonstrated that patients without recurrence within the first 3 months after ablation had a higher chance of "long-term clinical success" compared with those with early recurrence (95% vs 43%; P<.0001). Note that the mean follow-up period was 18.7 ± 7.2 months, and therefore the use of end point of "long-term clinical success" should be interpreted with caution. Importantly, however, the presence of structural heart disease was significantly associated with early recurrence in this study. More recently, Bazoukis and coworkers[51] similarly showed that early arrhythmia recurrence (within 3 months) was also associated with later recurrence (n = 38; mean follow-up period of 3.3 years).

### Late Gadolinium Enhancement by Cardiac MRI

There is increasing evidence regarding the utility of cardiac MRI (CMR) in predicting outcomes of catheter ablation. Fibrotic myocardial tissue has an expanded extracellular space, allowing for accumulation of gadolinium and therefore a higher signal intensity compared with healthy myocardium in T1-weighted MRI scans.[52,53] The DECAAF trial examined atrial tissue fibrosis estimation with delayed gadolinium enhancement and risk of AF recurrence. The unadjusted cumulative incidence of recurrent arrhythmia increased from 15.3% in patients with stage I fibrosis to 51.1% in those with stage IV fibrosis.[54] In addition, patients with no recurrence of AF following ablation showed a significantly lower burden of fibrosis in follow-up CMR scans, implying that patients with a greater burden of residual fibrosis should avoid repeat ablations unless no other options exist.[55]

Limitations to this approach exist. The spatial resolution of CMR scans is 1.2 to 1.5 mm (compared with an average atrial wall thickness of 2–4 mm), which increases the risk of incorrectly

characterizing surrounding tissue as LA wall.[56,57] Furthermore, more research is required to optimize understanding of the relationship between the voltage thresholds used for identifying fibrotic areas on voltage mapping and late gadolinium enhancement of CMR. Currently, voltage mapping by sampling electrical signals from atrial tissue is the gold standard for assessing and staging atrial fibrosis,[58] with an arbitrary threshold of a bipolar voltage less than or equal to 0.05 mV based on baseline noise in early mapping studies.[35] However, Jadidi and colleagues[59] showed that late gadolinium enhancement levels 5 standard deviations higher than the pool correlated with voltages of 0.38 ± 0.28 mV, indicating that 0.05 mV as a threshold may underestimate the degree of atrial fibrosis. Thus, further work is required to establish more specific cutoff voltages.

### Biomarkers

Several blood biomarkers have been shown to indicate risk of AF incidence and recurrence.[60] C-reactive protein has been investigated because of the role of the inflammatory milieu and oxidative stress in the induction of AF. A meta-analysis of seven heterogenous observational studies showed that higher baseline C-reactive protein levels was associated with a higher risk of recurrence after cardioversion.[61]

In addition, numerous biomarkers including high-sensitivity troponin, N-terminal pro-brain natriuretic peptide (NT-proBNP), and three fragments of vasoactive peptides (proadrenomedullin, copeptin, and CT-proendothelin-1) were studied in the GISSI-AF trial.[62] Higher levels of all biomarkers were shown to correlate with AF recurrence at 6 and 12 months in the 382 patients studied. However, there was a particularly significant association of NT-proBNP with median levels at 191 (interquartile range, 95–363) at baseline, 700 (402–1205) in those with recurrence at 6 months, and 560 (308–1051) in those with recurrence at 12 months (P<.0001). A meta-analysis including 10 studies on BNP and eight studies on NT-proBNP demonstrated a correlation between the levels of these two peptides and risk of AF recurrence, with standardized mean differences of 0.55 (95% CI, 0.26–0.84) and 0.96 (95% CI, 0.62–1.30), respectively.[63] However, these studies were mostly univariate analyses and therefore the role of additional confounding variables is unknown.

It should be noted, however, that current clinical guidelines do not delineate a role for biomarkers in the management of AF, or in determining the ideal management strategy for these patients.

## Left Atrial Volume and Sphericity

The recent multicenter LAGO-AF trial included 243 patients and used a three-dimensional model of the LA (mostly obtained with LA MR angiogram) to quantify LA volume and sphericity.[64] Adjusted Cox models identified paroxysmal AF (hazard ratio, 0.54; $P$ = .032) and LA sphericity (hazard ratio, 1.87; $P$ = .035) as independent markers of AF recurrence. The authors further developed a five-point LAGO score (AF phenotype, presence of structural heart disease, CHA2DS2-VASc $\leq$1, LA sphericity [$\geq$82.1% was considered spherical], and dilated LA [LA diameter >42 mm]). Patients with a low-risk score ($\leq$2 points) had a lower risk of recurrence at 3 years compared with those with a high-risk ($\geq$3 points) score (35% vs 82%; $P$<.001). Apart from necessitating LA MR angiogram, which is an added cost and may not be widely available, the study was limited by the assessment of recurrence with repeated 24-hour Holter monitors at unspecified time intervals, which may underestimate the degree of recurrence.

## Stage of Atrial Fibrillation

A systematic review by Balk and colleagues[65] in 2010 noted that 17 studies evaluated the type of AF (paroxysmal vs nonparoxysmal) and the risk of recurrence using multivariable analyses. Of these studies, only six showed that nonparoxysmal AF was an independent predictor of a higher rate of recurrence.[66–70] Meta-analyses examining AF recurrence rates by univariate analysis (31 studies) showed that persistent AF was associated with higher AF recurrence compared with paroxysmal AF (relative risk, 1.59; 95% CI, 1.38–1.82; $P$<.001).[65] However, these studies remain limited by the heterogeneity of methods used and small sample sizes.

## Other Comorbidities

A recent study by Arora and colleagues[71] in more than 37,000 patients demonstrated that predictors associated with AF recurrence (which the authors defined as readmission for AF or repeat ablation within 90 days of the initial ablation) included female sex, diabetes mellitus, chronic lung disease, and length of stay during initial ablation hospitalization of 2 days or longer. It should be noted that only 28.8% of patients in this study had a diagnosis of HF.

## MANAGEMENT OF PATIENTS WITH ATRIAL FIBRILLATION RECURRENCE

Management of patients with HF who have recurrence of AF following catheter ablation (**Fig. 1**)

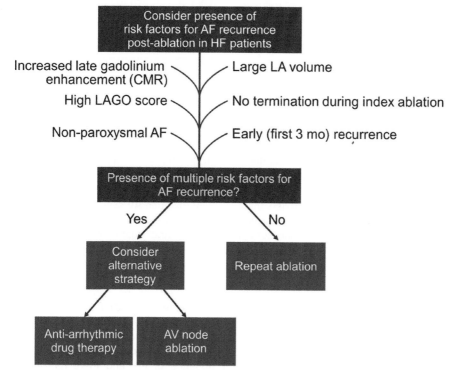

**Fig. 1.** Algorithm delineating predictors of AF recurrence and subsequent management of AF recurrence postablation. The LAGO score is a five-point score to identify the risk of AF recurrence postablation with points for AF phenotype (paroxysmal), presence of structural heart disease, CHA2DS2-VASc less than or equal to one, LA sphericity ($\geq$82.1% was considered spherical), and dilated LA (LA diameter >42 mm).

is challenging. Considerations include the risk and likely efficacy of repeat catheter ablation (based on the aforementioned predictive factors), previous tolerance of AADs, and whether they meet indications for additional therapies including AV nodal ablation and/or cardiac resynchronization therapy (CRT).

## Pharmacologic Therapy

Pharmacologic therapy can be trialled in patients at high risk of ablation failure, in those who decline further invasive treatments, or are deemed unlikely to benefit from additional ablation. Because of their arrhythmogenic potential, the choice of AAD therapy in patients with HFrEF and concomitant AF is limited to dofetilide, sotalol, or amiodarone, per the 2014 American Heart Association/American College of Cardiology guidelines.[72] Sotalol has negative inotropic effects in HF and sotalol and dofetilide have been associated with torsades de pointes, particularly in patients with renal insufficiency.[72] Sotalol can be used in some cases, as Plewan and coworkers[73] demonstrated efficacy in preventing AF recurrence in patients with a mean EF of 41 $\pm$ 5%, because of its β-blockade effect. However, in a retrospective analysis from 22 trials including 3135 patients receiving sotalol, HF was a factor predictive of torsades de pointes, and so caution should be exercised.[74] Class Ic agents (flecainide, propafenone) should be avoided in patients with HF because of their negative inotropic effects.[72]

The efficacy of dofetilide was demonstrated in the DIAMOND-CHF trial, which randomized 1518 patients with HF to dofetilide versus placebo. Dofetilide was more effective in maintaining sinus rhythm and reduced all-cause and HF hospitalizations (relative risk, 0.75 [0.63–0.89]).[75,76]

Amiodarone has been shown to effectively maintain sinus rhythm in patients with AF, although its efficacy is far from perfect (65% at 3 years).[3] A meta-analysis of 39 randomized controlled trials comparing multiple AADs including amiodarone, dronedarone, flecainide propafenone, and sotalol compared with placebo demonstrated that treatment with amiodarone had the highest probability of reducing AF recurrence (odds ratio [OR], 0.22; 95% CI, 0.16–0.29).[77] It should be noted, however, that use of dronedarone should be avoided in patients with an EF less than or equal to 35% because of increased mortality demonstrated in this group.[78] However, the use of amiodarone has been associated with multiple extracardiac toxicities, most notably pulmonary, hepatic, and endocrine (thyroid) effects. The same meta-analysis demonstrated that the use of amiodarone

was associated with the highest rates of experiencing adverse effects (OR, 2.41; 95% CI, 0.96–6.06) and treatment discontinuation caused by adverse events (OR, 2.91; 95% CI, 1.66–5.11), along with a trend toward increased mortality (OR, 2.17; 95% CI, 0.63–7.51).[77] The latter was further corroborated by the Sudden Cardiac Death in Heart Failure Trial (SCD-HeFT), performed in NYHA functional class II/III patients with an LVEF less than or equal to 35%, which demonstrated no difference in all-cause mortality when amiodarone was compared with implantable cardioverter-defibrillator (ICD) therapy, but did note an increase in noncardiac mortality in NYHA functional class II patients.[79] The proportion of patients who had previously undergone catheter ablation is unclear in DIAMOND-CHF and SCD-HeFT, although the latter did exclude patients who had previously undergone AV nodal ablation.

## Nonpharmacologic Therapies

In patients in whom rate control with AADs or catheter ablation has failed, AV node ablation (AVNA) is an option, although this is often a last resort because it necessitates permanent pacemaker implantation and the patient will be pacemaker dependent. This has documented efficacy and has been shown to reduce physician office visits episodes of HF, and subsequent use of AADs including in older patient cohorts.[80–82] A meta-analysis comprising more than 6700 patients showed improvement of symptoms and quality of life with AVNA compared with medical therapy with no difference in all-cause mortality.[83] However, a subgroup analysis of 116 patients with systolic dysfunction showed that these patients had a significant improvement in EF after AVNA (+4% greater; 95% CI, 3.11–4.89). Furthermore, studies have shown that patients with paroxysmal AF derive more benefit from dual-chamber pacemakers with mode-switching capabilities because they maintain AV synchrony during times of sinus rhythm (compared with single-chamber pacemakers and dual-chamber pacemakers without mode-switching capabilities).[84,85]

Right ventricular (RV) pacing alone can result in electrical dyssynchrony, which can have detrimental effects on cardiac function and further potentiate HF.[86] CRT can help to mitigate RV pacing-induced cardiomyopathy and potentially improve EF and symptoms. In addition, CRT is indicated in certain patients with HF, even in the absence of AF, and there has been interest in determining whether patients with HF would automatically benefit from CRT following AVNA. The PAVE trial randomized 184 patients with AF and

HF (83% NYHA functional class II or III) to either standard RV pacing or CRT pacing following AVNA.[87] Patients who received CRT had improved 6-minute-walk distances and EFs at 6 months, and subgroup analysis showed that greater improvement was noted in patients with NYHA functional class II/III symptoms or EF less than or equal to 45%. The BLOCK-HF trial randomized 691 patients with NYHA functional class I/II/III HF and LVEF less than or equal to 50% to either RV pacing or CRT following AVNA and showed that patients in the CRT group had a lower incidence of the composite end point of all-cause mortality, urgent care visit for HF requiring intravenous therapy, or greater than or equal to 15% increase in LV end-systolic volume index (hazard ratio, 0.74; 95% CI, 0.6–0.9).[88]

The RAFT trial, which included a subgroup analysis of 229 patients with AF, compared CRT plus ICD (CRT-D) with ICD therapy alone. There was no difference in death or HF hospitalizations between the two groups.[89] It should be noted, however, that only 34.3% of CRT patients had at least 95% biventricular pacing during the first 6 months. A study of 162 patients with AF who had undergone CRT placement for conventional HF indications (LVEF ≤35%, NYHA functional class ≥II, and a QRS duration >120 milliseconds) showed that only patients who had undergone concomitant AVNA exhibited significant improvement in EF, reverse remodeling, and exercise tolerance.[90] This underscored the notion that AVNA may be necessary to abolish intrinsic dyssynchronous conduction that can occur with rapid conduction down the AV node in patients with AF, to maximally benefit from CRT. This was confirmed in a study of approximately 37,000 patients who underwent remote monitoring of their CRT devices, with patients who had greater than or equal to 99.6% biventricular pacing experiencing a 24% decrease in mortality.[91] The results of these trials suggest that patients with symptomatic systolic dysfunction or those who deteriorate after RV pacing may benefit from CRT therapy following AVNA.[92]

## SUMMARY

Patients with AF, and especially those with concomitant HF who undergo catheter ablation, remain at high risk of recurrence. A multifactorial approach can be used to try to determine which patients are at higher risk of recurrence (including such parameters as LA volume, late gadolinium enhancement by CMR, the type of AF, and novel risk scoring methods using measures, such as LA sphericity). It is also important to consider the role of nonpharmacologic options, such as AVNA and CRT, in select patients as additional treatment options beyond repeat ablation and AAD therapy.

## REFERENCES

1. Miyasaka Y, Barnes ME, Bailey KR, et al. Mortality trends in patients diagnosed with first atrial fibrillation: a 21-year community-based study. J Am Coll Cardiol 2007;49(9):986–92.
2. Kirchhof P, Benussi S, Kotecha D, et al. 2016 ESC Guidelines for the management of atrial fibrillation developed in collaboration with EACTS. Eur Heart J 2016;37(38):2893–962.
3. Zimetbaum P. Antiarrhythmic drug therapy for atrial fibrillation. Circulation 2012;125(2):381–9.
4. Chen MS, Marrouche NF, Khaykin Y, et al. Pulmonary vein isolation for the treatment of atrial fibrillation in patients with impaired systolic function. J Am Coll Cardiol 2004;43(6):1004–9.
5. MacDonald MR, Connelly DT, Hawkins NM, et al. Radiofrequency ablation for persistent atrial fibrillation in patients with advanced heart failure and severe left ventricular systolic dysfunction: a randomised controlled trial. Heart 2011;97(9):740–7.
6. Di Biase L, Mohanty P, Mohanty S, et al. Ablation vs. amiodarone for treatment of persistent atrial fibrillation in patients with congestive heart failure and an implanted device: results from the AATAC multicenter randomized trial. Circulation 2016;133(17):1637–44.
7. Wilton SB, Fundytus A, Ghali WA, et al. Meta-analysis of the effectiveness and safety of catheter ablation of atrial fibrillation in patients with versus without left ventricular systolic dysfunction. Am J Cardiol 2010;106(9):1284–91.
8. Dagres N, Varounis C, Gaspar T, et al. Catheter ablation for atrial fibrillation in patients with left ventricular systolic dysfunction. A systematic review and meta-analysis. J Card Fail 2011;17(11):964–70.
9. Anselmino M, Matta M, D'ascenzo F, et al. Catheter ablation of atrial fibrillation in patients with left ventricular systolic dysfunction: a systematic review and meta-analysis. Circ Arrhythm Electrophysiol 2014;7(6):1011–8.
10. Ganesan AN, Nandal S, Lüker J, et al. Catheter ablation of atrial fibrillation in patients with concomitant left ventricular impairment: a systematic review of efficacy and effect on ejection fraction. Heart Lung Circ 2015;24(3):270–80.
11. Marrouche NF, Brachmann J, Andresen D, et al. Catheter ablation for atrial fibrillation with heart failure. N Engl J Med 2018;378(5):417–27.
12. Packer DL, Mark DB, Robb RA, et al. Catheter ablation versus antiarrhythmic drug therapy for atrial fibrillation (CABANA) trial: study rationale and design. Am Heart J 2018;199:192–9.

13. Kobza R, Hindricks G, Tanner H, et al. Late recurrent arrhythmias after ablation of atrial fibrillation: incidence, mechanisms, and treatment. Heart Rhythm 2004;1(6):676–83.

14. Al-Hijji MA, Deshmukh AJ, Yao X, et al. Trends and predictors of repeat catheter ablation for atrial fibrillation. Am Heart J 2016;171(1):48–55.

15. Bunch TJ, Cutler MJ. Is pulmonary vein isolation still the cornerstone in atrial fibrillation ablation? J Thorac Dis 2015;7(2):132.

16. Malhi N, Hawkins NM, Andrade JG, et al. Catheter ablation of atrial fibrillation in heart failure with reduced ejection fraction. J Cardiovasc Electrophysiol 2018;29(7):1049–58.

17. Casaclang-Verzosa G, Gersh BJ, Tsang TS. Structural and functional remodeling of the left atrium: clinical and therapeutic implications for atrial fibrillation. J Am Coll Cardiol 2008;51(1):1–11.

18. Stambler BS, Fenelon G, Shepard RK, et al. Characterization of sustained atrial tachycardia in dogs with rapid ventricular pacing-induced heart failure. J Cardiovasc Electrophysiol 2003;14(5):499–507.

19. De Vos CB, Pisters R, Nieuwlaat R, et al. Progression from paroxysmal to persistent atrial fibrillation: clinical correlates and prognosis. J Am Coll Cardiol 2010;55(8):725–31.

20. Zhang Z, Letsas KP, Zhang N, et al. Linear ablation following pulmonary vein isolation in patients with atrial fibrillation: a meta-analysis. Pacing Clin Electrophysiol 2016;39(6):623–30.

21. Latchamsetty R, Morady F. Complex fractionated atrial electrograms: a worthwhile target for ablation of atrial fibrillation? Circ Arrhythm Electrophysiol 2011;4(2):117–8.

22. Buch E, Share M, Tung R, et al. Long-term clinical outcomes of focal impulse and rotor modulation for treatment of atrial fibrillation: a multicenter experience. Heart Rhythm 2016;13(3):636–41.

23. Nery PB, Thornhill R, Nair GM, et al. Scar-based catheter ablation for persistent atrial fibrillation. Curr Opin Cardiol 2017;32(1):1–9.

24. Zhao Y, Di Biase L, Trivedi C, et al. Importance of non–pulmonary vein triggers ablation to achieve long-term freedom from paroxysmal atrial fibrillation in patients with low ejection fraction. Heart Rhythm 2016;13(1):141–9.

25. Dixit S, Marchlinski FE, Lin D, et al. Randomized ablation strategies for the treatment of persistent atrial fibrillation: RASTA study. Circ Arrhythm Electrophysiol 2012;5(2):287–94.

26. Dzau VJ, Colucci WS, Hollenberg NK, et al. Relation of the renin-angiotensin-aldosterone system to clinical state in congestive heart failure. Circulation 1981;63(3):645–51.

27. Jayachandran JV, Sih HJ, Winkle W, et al. Atrial fibrillation produced by prolonged rapid atrial pacing is associated with heterogeneous changes in atrial sympathetic innervation. Circulation 2000;101(10):1185–91.

28. Nguyen BL, Fishbein MC, Chen LS, et al. Histopathological substrate for chronic atrial fibrillation in humans. Heart Rhythm 2009;6(4):454–60.

29. Tan AY, Zhou S, Ogawa M, et al. Neural mechanisms of paroxysmal atrial fibrillation and paroxysmal atrial tachycardia in ambulatory canines. Circulation 2008;118(9):916–25.

30. Chen P-S, Chen LS, Fishbein MC, et al. Role of the autonomic nervous system in atrial fibrillation: pathophysiology and therapy. Circ Res 2014;114(9):1500–15.

31. Chen LY, Chung MK, Allen LA, et al. Atrial fibrillation burden: moving beyond atrial fibrillation as a binary entity: a scientific statement from the American Heart Association. Circulation 2018;137(20):e623–44.

32. Black-Maier E, Ren X, Steinberg BA, et al. Catheter ablation of atrial fibrillation in patients with heart failure and preserved ejection fraction. Heart rhythm 2018;15(5):651–7.

33. Njoku A, Kannabhiran M, Arora R, et al. Left atrial volume predicts atrial fibrillation recurrence after radiofrequency ablation: a meta-analysis. Europace 2017;20(1):33–42.

34. Zhuang Y, Yong Y-H, Chen M-l. Updating the evidence for the effect of radiofrequency catheter ablation on left atrial volume and function in patients with atrial fibrillation: a meta-analysis. JRSM Open 2014;5(3). 2054270414521185.

35. Sanders P, Morton JB, Davidson NC, et al. Electrical remodeling of the atria in congestive heart failure: electrophysiological and electroanatomic mapping in humans. Circulation 2003;108(12):1461–8.

36. Li D, Fareh S, Leung TK, et al. Promotion of atrial fibrillation by heart failure in dogs: atrial remodeling of a different sort. Circulation 1999;100(1):87–95.

37. Verma A, Wazni OM, Marrouche NF, et al. Pre-existent left atrial scarring in patients undergoing pulmonary vein antrum isolation: an independent predictor of procedural failure. J Am Coll Cardiol 2005;45(2):285–92.

38. Lu T-M, Tai C-T, Hsieh M-H, et al. Electrophysiologic characteristics in initiation of paroxysmal atrial fibrillation from a focal area. J Am Coll Cardiol 2001;37(6):1658–64.

39. Verheule S, Sato T, Everett T 4th, et al. Increased vulnerability to atrial fibrillation in transgenic mice with selective atrial fibrosis caused by overexpression of TGF-β1. Circ Res 2004;94(11):1458–65.

40. Peters DC, Wylie JV, Hauser TH, et al. Recurrence of atrial fibrillation correlates with the extent of postprocedural late gadolinium enhancement: a pilot study. JACC Cardiovasc Imaging 2009;2(3):308–16.

41. Wylie JV Jr, Peters DC, Essebag V, et al. Left atrial function and scar after catheter ablation of atrial fibrillation. Heart rhythm 2008;5(5):656–62.

42. Reddy YN, El Sabbagh A, Packer D, et al. Evaluation of shortness of breath after atrial fibrillation ablation—is there a stiff left atrium? Heart rhythm 2018; 15(6):930–5.

43. O'Neill MD, Wright M, Knecht S, et al. Long-term follow-up of persistent atrial fibrillation ablation using termination as a procedural endpoint. Eur Heart J 2009;30(9):1105–12.

44. Park YM, CHOI JI, Lim HE, et al. Is pursuit of termination of atrial fibrillation during catheter ablation of great value in patients with longstanding persistent atrial fibrillation? J Cardiovasc Electrophysiol 2012; 23(10):1051–8.

45. Ma X, Zhang X, Guo W. Factors to predict recurrence of atrial fibrillation in patients with hypertension. Clin Cardiol 2009;32(5):264–8.

46. Bollmann A, Kanuru N, McTeague K, et al. Frequency analysis of human atrial fibrillation using the surface electrocardiogram and its response to ibutilide. Am J Cardiol 1998;81(12):1439–45.

47. Langberg J, Bollmann A, Pena E, et al. Frequency analysis of the ECG during atrial fibrillation predicts recurrence after cardioversion. Pacing Clin Electrophysiol 1998;21:858.

48. Fynn SP, Todd DM, Hobbs WJC, et al. Role of dispersion of atrial refractoriness in the recurrence of clinical atrial fibrillation. A manifestation of atrial electrical remodelling in humans? Eur Heart J 2001;22(19):1822–34.

49. Cai L, Yin Y, Ling Z, et al. Predictors of late recurrence of atrial fibrillation after catheter ablation. Int J Cardiol 2013;164(1):82–7.

50. Bertaglia E, Stabile G, Senatore G, et al. Predictive value of early atrial tachyarrhythmias recurrence after circumferential anatomical pulmonary vein ablation. Pacing Clin Electrophysiol 2005;28(5):366–71.

51. Bazoukis G, Letsas KP, Tse G, et al. Predictors of arrhythmia recurrence in patients with heart failure undergoing left atrial ablation for atrial fibrillation. Clin Cardiol 2018;41(1):63–7.

52. Burstein B, Nattel S. Atrial fibrosis: mechanisms and clinical relevance in atrial fibrillation. J Am Coll Cardiol 2008;51(8):802–9.

53. Kim RJ, Chen E-L, Judd RM. Myocardial Gd-DTPA kinetics determine MRI contrast enhancement and reflect the extent and severity of myocardial injury after acute reperfused infarction. Circulation 1996; 94(12):3318–26.

54. Marrouche NF, Wilber D, Hindricks G, et al. Association of atrial tissue fibrosis identified by delayed enhancement MRI and atrial fibrillation catheter ablation: the DECAAF study. JAMA 2014;311(5):498–506.

55. Gal P, Marrouche NF. Magnetic resonance imaging of atrial fibrosis: redefining atrial fibrillation to a syndrome. Eur Heart J 2015;38(1):14–9.

56. Kawel N, Turkbey EB, Carr JJ, et al. Normal left ventricular myocardial thickness for middle-aged and older subjects with steady-state free precession cardiac magnetic resonance: the multi-ethnic study of atherosclerosis. Circ Cardiovasc Imaging 2012; 5(4):500–8.

57. Appelbaum E, Manning WJ. Left atrial fibrosis by late gadolinium enhancement cardiovascular magnetic resonance predicts recurrence of atrial fibrillation after pulmonary vein isolation: do you see what I see? Circ Arrhythm Electrophysiol 2014;7(1):2–4.

58. Kottkamp H. Human atrial fibrillation substrate: towards a specific fibrotic atrial cardiomyopathy. Eur Heart J 2013;34(35):2731–8.

59. Jadidi AS, Cochet H, Shah AJ, et al. Inverse relationship between fractionated electrograms and atrial fibrosis in persistent atrial fibrillation: combined magnetic resonance imaging and high-density mapping. J Am Coll Cardiol 2013;62(9):802–12.

60. Vizzardi E, Curnis A, Latini MG, et al. Risk factors for atrial fibrillation recurrence: a literature review. J Cardiovasc Med 2014;15(3):235–53.

61. Liu T, Li G, Li L, et al. Association between C-reactive protein and recurrence of atrial fibrillation after successful electrical cardioversion: a meta-analysis. J Am Coll Cardiol 2007;49(15):1642–8.

62. Latini R, Masson S, Pirelli S, et al. Circulating cardiovascular biomarkers in recurrent atrial fibrillation: data from the GISSI-atrial fibrillation trial. J Intern Med 2011;269(2):160–71.

63. Zhang Y, Chen A, Song L, et al. Association between baseline natriuretic peptides and atrial fibrillation recurrence after catheter ablation. Int Heart J 2016;57(2):183–9.

64. Bisbal F, Alarcón F, Ferrero-de-Loma-Osorio A, et al. Left atrial geometry and outcome of atrial fibrillation ablation: results from the multicentre LAGO-AF study. Eur Heart J Cardiovasc Imaging 2018;19(9): 1002–9.

65. Balk EM, Garlitski AC, Alsheikh-Ali AA, et al. Predictors of atrial fibrillation recurrence after radiofrequency catheter ablation: a systematic review. J Cardiovasc Electrophysiol 2010;21(11):1208–16.

66. Cheema A, Vasamreddy CR, Dalal D, et al. Long-term single procedure efficacy of catheter ablation of atrial fibrillation. J Interv Card Electrophysiol 2006;15(3):145–55.

67. Themistoclakis S, Schweikert RA, Saliba WI, et al. Clinical predictors and relationship between early and late atrial tachyarrhythmias after pulmonary vein antrum isolation. Heart Rhythm 2008;5(5):679–85.

68. Pappone C, Manguso F, Vicedomini G, et al. Prevention of iatrogenic atrial tachycardia after ablation of atrial fibrillation: a prospective randomized study comparing circumferential pulmonary vein ablation with a modified approach. Circulation 2004; 110(19):3036–42.

69. Richter B, Gwechenberger M, Filzmoser P, et al. Is inducibility of atrial fibrillation after radio frequency

ablation really a relevant prognostic factor? Eur Heart J 2006;27(21):2553–9.

70. Essebag V, Baldessin F, Reynolds MR, et al. Non-inducibility post-pulmonary vein isolation achieving exit block predicts freedom from atrial fibrillation. Eur Heart J 2005;26(23):2550–5.

71. Arora S, Lahewala S, Tripathi B, et al. Causes and predictors of readmission in patients with atrial fibrillation undergoing catheter ablation: a national population-based cohort study. J Am Heart Assoc 2018;7(12) [pii:e009294].

72. January CT, Wann LS, Alpert JS, et al. 2014 AHA/ACC/HRS guideline for the management of patients with atrial fibrillation: executive summary: a report of the American College of Cardiology/American Heart Association Task Force on practice guidelines and the Heart Rhythm Society. J Am Coll Cardiol 2014; 64(21):2246–80.

73. Plewan A, Lehmann G, Ndrepepa G, et al. Maintenance of sinus rhythm after electrical cardioversion of persistent atrial fibrillation. Sotalol vs bisoprolol. Eur Heart J 2001;22(16):1504–10.

74. Lehmann MH, Hardy S, Archibald D, et al. Sex difference in risk of torsade de pointes with d, l-sotalol. Circulation 1996;94(10):2535–41.

75. Pedersen OD, Bagger H, Keller N, et al. Efficacy of dofetilide in the treatment of atrial fibrillation-flutter in patients with reduced left ventricular function: a Danish investigations of arrhythmia and mortality on dofetilide (diamond) substudy. Circulation 2001; 104(3):292–6.

76. Dixit S, Gerstenfeld EP, Callans DJ, et al. Comparison of cool tip versus 8-mm tip catheter in achieving electrical isolation of pulmonary veins for long-term control of atrial fibrillation: a prospective randomized pilot study. J Cardiovasc Electrophysiol 2006;17(10):1074–9.

77. Freemantle N, Lafuente-Lafuente C, Mitchell S, et al. Mixed treatment comparison of dronedarone, amiodarone, sotalol, flecainide, and propafenone, for the management of atrial fibrillation. Europace 2011; 13(3):329–45.

78. Køber L, Torp-Pedersen C, McMurray JJ, et al. Increased mortality after dronedarone therapy for severe heart failure. N Engl J Med 2008;358(25): 2678–87.

79. Packer DL, Prutkin JM, Hellkamp AS, et al. Impact of implantable cardioverter-defibrillator, amiodarone, and placebo on the mode of death in stable patients with heart failure: analysis from the sudden cardiac death in heart failure trial. Circulation 2009;120(22): 2170–6.

80. Scheinman MM, Huang S. The 1998 NASPE prospective catheter ablation registry. Pacing Clin Electrophysiol 2000;23(6):1020–8.

81. Fitzpatrick AP, Kourouyan HD, Siu A, et al. Quality of life and outcomes after radiofrequency His-bundle catheter ablation and permanent pacemaker implantation: impact of treatment in paroxysmal and established atrial fibrillation. Am Heart J 1996; 131(3):499–507.

82. Ozcan C, Jahangir A, Friedman PA, et al. Long-term survival after ablation of the atrioventricular node and implantation of a permanent pacemaker in patients with atrial fibrillation. N Engl J Med 2001; 344(14):1043–51.

83. Chatterjee NA, Upadhyay GA, Ellenbogen KA, et al. Atrioventricular nodal ablation in atrial fibrillation: a meta-analysis and systematic review. Circ Arrhythm Electrophysiol 2012;5(1):68–76.

84. Marshall HJ, Harris ZI, Griffith MJ, et al. Prospective randomized study of ablation and pacing versus medical therapy for paroxysmal atrial fibrillation: effects of pacing mode and mode-switch algorithm. Circulation 1999;99(12):1587–92.

85. Kamalvand K, Tan K, Kotsakis A, et al. Is mode switching beneficial? A randomized study in patients with paroxysmal atrial tachyarrhythmias. J Am Coll Cardiol 1997;30(2):496–504.

86. Bank AJ, Gage RM, Burns KV. Right ventricular pacing, mechanical dyssynchrony, and heart failure. J Cardiovasc Transl Res 2012;5(2):219–31.

87. Doshi RN, Daoud EG, Fellows C, et al. Left ventricular-based cardiac stimulation post AV nodal ablation E valuation (The PAVE Study). J Cardiovasc Electrophysiol 2005;16(11):1160–5.

88. Curtis AB, Worley SJ, Adamson PB, et al. Biventricular pacing for atrioventricular block and systolic dysfunction. N Engl J Med 2013;368(17):1585–93.

89. Healey JS, Hohnloser SH, Exner DV, et al. Cardiac resynchronization therapy in patients with permanent atrial fibrillation: results from the Resynchronization for Ambulatory Heart Failure Trial (RAFT). Circ Heart Fail 2012;5(5):566–70.

90. Gasparini M, Auricchio A, Regoli F, et al. Four-year efficacy of cardiac resynchronization therapy on exercise tolerance and disease progression: the importance of performing atrioventricular junction ablation in patients with atrial fibrillation. J Am Coll Cardiol 2006;48(4):734–43.

91. Hayes DL, Boehmer JP, Day JD, et al. Cardiac resynchronization therapy and the relationship of percent biventricular pacing to symptoms and survival. Heart Rhythm 2011;8(9):1469–75.

92. Leon AR, Greenberg JM, Kanuru N, et al. Cardiac resynchronization in patients with congestive heart failure and chronic atrial fibrillation: effect of upgrading to biventricular pacing after chronic right ventricular pacing. J Am Coll Cardiol 2002;39(8):1258–63.

# Should His Bundle Pacing Be Preferred over Cardiac Resynchronization Therapy Following Atrioventricular Junction Ablation?

Zak Loring, MD[a,b],*, Albert Y. Sun, MD[a,c]

## KEYWORDS

- His bundle pacing • Biventricular pacemaker • Cardiac resynchronization therapy • Atrial fibrillation
- Catheter ablation • Heart failure

## KEY POINTS

- Atrial fibrillation (AF) and heart failure (HF) are associated with high morbidity and mortality.
- Atrioventricular junction (AVJ) ablation with pacemaker implantation can be used in patients with incessant AF with rapid ventricular rate.
- The optimal choice of pacing strategy for patients with HF after AVJ ablation is unknown.
- His bundle pacing (HBP) and biventricular (BiV) pacing both offer more physiologic activation compared with right ventricle only pacemakers.
- This review describes the benefits and drawbacks of HBP and BiV pacing in HF patients after AVJ ablation.

## INTRODUCTION

Atrial fibrillation (AF) is a common arrhythmia with increasing prevalence[1] and is associated with frequent hospitalizations and high treatment costs.[2] When AF occurs in the setting of heart failure (HF), the deleterious effects are magnified. Although the loss of atrial "kick" and atrioventricular (AV) synchrony both contribute to this acquired morbidity, perhaps the most dramatic detrimental hemodynamic effects occur in the setting of AF with rapid ventricular rates (RVR). Rate control strategies in this scenario can be challenging because of the negative inotropic effects of some pharmacologic agents as well as subsequent symptomatic bradycardia (eg, tachycardia-bradycardia syndrome).[3] Pharmacologic rhythm control agents are limited to dofetilide and amiodarone in patients with structural heart disease and reduced left ventricular ejection fraction (LVEF).[3] Catheter ablation procedures have been shown to improve outcomes in patients with heart failure and reduced ejection fraction (HFrEF)[4,5]; however, the single procedure success rates of catheter ablation are lower in patients with HFrEF and persistent AF and can require multiple procedures.[6,7]

Creation of iatrogenic heart block via catheter ablation of the atrioventricular junction (AVJ) with pacemaker implantation can achieve complete,

Disclosure Statement: The authors have no relevant disclosures.
a Division of Cardiology, Section of Electrophysiology, Duke University Medical Center, 2301 Erwin Road, Durham, NC 27710, USA; b Duke Clinical Research Institute, 200 Morris St, Durham, NC 27701, USA; c Division of Cardiology, Section of Electrophysiology, Durham VA Medical Center, 508 Fulton Street, Durham, NC 27705, USA
* Corresponding author. Duke University Medical Center, 2301 Erwin Road, DUMC 3845, Durham, NC 27710.
E-mail address: zak.loring@duke.edu

Cardiol Clin 37 (2019) 231–240
https://doi.org/10.1016/j.ccl.2019.01.006
0733-8651/19/© 2019 Elsevier Inc. All rights reserved.

although irreversible, rate control in patients with incessant AF with RVR,[8] and incidentally was the first condition in which catheter ablation in humans was performed.[9] Patients undergoing AVJ ablation with normal ejection fractions (EF) are given single-site right ventricular (RV) pacemakers as standard of care; in patients with reduced EFs, however, randomized trials demonstrated that cardiac resynchronization therapy (CRT) via biventricular (BiV) pacemaker systems results in improved clinical outcomes.[10] Given the high pacing burden after AVJ ablation, pacing in a more physiologic way is preferred to reduce the risk of pacemaker-induced cardiomyopathy due to frequent RV pacing.[11] BiV pacemakers using coronary sinus (CS) lead placement have been the mainstay of physiologic pacing in the past; however, His bundle pacing (HBP) has emerged as an alternative and promising pacing method that mimics physiologic activation patterns by directly stimulating the patient's native conduction system.[12] Ongoing clinical trials, such as the His-SYNC trial (Clincialtrials.gov; NCT02700425), have been comparing clinical outcomes between these 2 strategies in HF patients, because the superior choice is not currently known. This review describes the benefits and drawbacks of BiV pacing and HBP in the setting of HF and AVJ ablation.

## BIVENTRICULAR PACEMAKERS

Compared with single-site RV-only pacing, BiV pacemakers provide more physiologic pacing by coordinating activation of the septum (via an RV lead) and lateral wall (via a CS lead) of the left ventricle (LV), allowing for a more synchronous LV contraction. Utilization of BiV pacing in patients with HF and left bundle branch block (LBBB) has been shown to improve clinical outcomes in multiple large clinical trials, and since being approved by the Food and Drug Administration in 2001, the use of BiV pacing has steadily increased over time.[13–15]

### Biventricular Pacemakers in Atrioventricular Block

The LV activation and contraction pattern resulting from RV-only pacing is similar to the patterns seen in LBBB, prompting investigators to hypothesize that BiV pacing may be superior to RV-only pacing in patients anticipated to have a high pacing burden.[16] The Biventricular versus Right Ventricular Pacing in Heart Failure Patients with Atrioventricular Block (BLOCK-HF) trial demonstrated that in patients with AV block, New York Heart Association (NYHA) symptom class I–III HF and an LVEF ≤50%, patients randomized to BiV pacing had fewer adverse clinical outcomes, more LV

remodeling, and more symptomatic improvement compared with patients randomized to RV-only pacing.[17–19] After the release of the BLOCK-HF trial, preliminary results from the Biventricular Pacing for Atrioventricular Block to Prevent Cardiac Desynchronization (BioPace) trial were reported evaluating the difference in death or HF hospitalization between patients with AV block and HF randomized to BiV pacing versus RV-only pacing.[20] The BioPace trial had a similar patient composition to BLOCK-HF but enrolled patients with less severe AV block (first- and second-degree AV block as well as patients with AF and a ventricular rate ≤60 beats/min) and higher average EFs (55% vs 40%). The results showed a trend toward superiority of BiV pacing that did not reach statistical significance, including in the subgroup of patients with EF less than 50%.[21] A systematic review of studies comparing BiV pacing or HBP (physiologic pacing) to RV-only pacing in patients without severe LV systolic dysfunction (EF >35%) found that patients with EF greater than 35% but ≤52% were more likely to benefit from physiologic pacing compared with RV-only pacing.[22] The most recent guidelines provide a IIa recommendation for use of pacing methods that maintain physiologic ventricular activation (ie, BiV pacing or HBP) in patients with an LVEF between 36% and 50% who are expected to require ventricular pacing more than 40% of the time.[23] These studies and guidelines support the superiority of physiologic pacing over RV-only pacing in patients with AV block and reduced EF.

### Biventricular Pacemakers after Atrioventricular Junction Ablation

Multiple studies have evaluated the effectiveness of BiV pacing in the setting of AVJ ablation. The post-AV nodal evaluation study randomized 184 patients undergoing AVJ ablation for AF with RVR to BiV pacing or RV-only pacing and evaluated 6-minute walk distances, quality of life, and LVEF at 6 months' follow-up.[10] Patients randomized to BiV pacing had better 6-minute walk distances and LVEF improvement compared with patients randomized to RV-only pacing. In addition, patients with LVEF ≤45% had the greatest improvement in 6-minute walk distances. The Ablate and Pace in Atrial Fibrillation (APAF) trial also compared BiV pacing to RV-only pacing in 186 patients undergoing AVJ ablation and showed that BiV pacing was associated with fewer HF deaths, HF hospitalization, or worsening HF symptoms compared with RV-only pacing.[24]

BiV pacing was designed to normalize LV activation in patients with underlying dyssynchrony;

however, in patients without significant electrical dyssynchrony at baseline, it can *cause* iatrogenic dyssynchrony.[25] Patients with narrow QRS complexes (<120 milliseconds) have been shown not to respond to BiV pacing, and BiV pacing may be harmful in these patients, leading to increased mortality.[26] Consistent with the possibility of harm, the Evaluation of Resynchronization Therapy for Heart Failure trial evaluating BiV pacing in patients with HF and a QRS duration less than 120 milliseconds was stopped by the Data Safety and Monitoring Board over safety concerns.[27] A meta-analysis also suggested a signal toward harm with use of BiV pacing in patients with QRS duration less than 130 milliseconds.[28] Although these studies were not done in patients with AV block or those undergoing AVJ ablation, they raise concerns about the efficacy of BiV pacing in patients without underling conduction disease. The APAF investigators conducted another trial to investigate the effectiveness of AVJ ablation and BiV pacing in patients with narrow QRS complexes (≤110 milliseconds) to better understand this issue. The Ablate and Pace in Atrial Fibrillation plus Cardiac Resynchronization Therapy trial randomized 102 patients with AF, narrow QRS complexes (≤110 milliseconds), and at least one HF hospitalization in the previous year to either AVJ ablation and BiV pacing or pharmacologic rate control.[29] AVJ ablation and BiV pacing resulted in lower rates of HF death, HF hospitalization, or worsening HF symptoms compared with pharmacologic rate control. The results of this trial suggest that BiV pacing after AVJ ablation is an effective strategy even in the absence of underlying conduction disease.

## Hemodynamic Effects of Biventricular Pacing

Ventricular activation in BiV pacing results in as many as 3 independent wave fronts (RV pacing lead, LV pacing lead, and any intrinsic conduction). Canine studies have compared total activation times (TAT) and LV contraction (as measured by LV dP/dT [first derivative of LV pressure]) during atrial pacing (simulating native conduction) and multiple combinations of A-RV and A-LV pacing intervals. BiV pacing resulted in higher LV dP/dT and lower TAT than RV-pacing at all tested AV intervals.[30] The hemodynamic effects of different pacing patterns have also been studied in patients with HF. A study of 11 HF patients with preexisting BBB compared LV dP/dT in atrial pacing (similar activation to RV-only pacing given preexisting BBB), BiV pacing, and LV-only pacing. BiV and LV-only pacing resulted in higher stroke volumes and dP/dT than the asymmetric activation seen

in atrial pacing with underlying LBBB.[31] These studies demonstrate that the synchronous activation resulting from BiV pacing results in superior LV mechanical function compared with asymmetric activation seen in RV-only pacing.

### Challenges with Biventricular Pacemakers

Although the outcomes for BiV after AVJ ablation appear to be superior to RV-only pacing, the need for a CS lead placement increases the complexity of implantation, fails in some patients, and can make device extraction more challenging. A systematic review comparing complications between dual-chamber implantable cardioverter-defibrillator and BiV devices revealed that implantation success in BiV devices was significantly lower (98.9% vs 92.5%) with higher rates of lead dislodgement during follow-up (5.9% vs 1.8%).[32] BiV devices also introduced additional risk with CS lead implantation, resulting in coronary venous complications in 2.0% of cases.[32] If lead extraction is necessary (eg, for systemic infection), CS lead extraction presents unique challenges due to the complexity of the anatomy, and postextraction venous occlusion can limit reimplantation options.[33] Although major complications with lead extraction are rare (approximately 1.8%), low LVEF and higher NYHA class are associated with higher risk of major complication and mortality, respectively.[34]

## HIS BUNDLE PACEMAKERS

Pacing the heart via the His bundle takes advantage of the patient's intrinsic conduction system to allow for activation most similar to patients' naturally occurring myocardial activation pattern. It was first described in a canine model 1967 by Scherlag and colleagues,[35] whereby Teflon-coated stainless steel wires were inserted into the His bundle through the lateral atrial wall and showed that pacing from this site produced a QRS complex that was indistinguishable from the morphology during sinus rhythm or atrial pacing. Scherlag and colleagues[36] were subsequently able to demonstrate His bundle recordings in humans using a catheter-based approach. The first permanent HBP in humans was described in 2000 in a study of 18 patients being treated for refractory AF with RVR with AVJ ablation in which His bundle stimulation was successful in 14 of the patients, and permanent HBP using a fixed screw-in lead was successfully achieved in 12 patients.[12] With the ability to chronically pace the His bundle via permanent pacemakers, further investigations of HBP as a means of achieving CRT were pursued.

### His Bundle Pacing in Atrioventricular Block

Given the physiologic activation patterns achievable with HBP, it is an attractive therapeutic solution for patients presenting with AV block. A randomized, double-blinded, crossover study compared HBP to RV-only pacing in patients with AV block, narrow QRS complexes (<120 milliseconds), and preserved LVEF (>40%). The study showed that HBP was successful in 85% of patients and achieved higher postintervention LVEF compared with RV-only pacing.[37]

One might expect AV block, particularly block due to infranodal disease, may not be as responsive to HBP. However, microscopic examination of the His bundle supported the previously postulated theory of functional longitudinal dissociation of the His bundle.[38,39] This theory purported that the fibers within the His bundle were predestined for the bundle branches and that proximal lesions could result in bundle branch blocks that could be overcome by pacing the His bundle distal or adjacent to the site of block. Indeed, early pacing studies demonstrated that HBP could overcome LBBB, previously thought to be due to conduction disease distal to the His bundle.[40] A study of patients referred for pacemaker evaluated HBP outcomes regardless of type of AV block (84 patients had narrow QRS, 98 patients had wide QRS complexes).[41] Successful HBP was achieved in 73% of patients (44 of the 84 patients with narrow QRS, 15 of the 98 with wide QRS complex), suggesting that although some patients with wide QRS are correctable with HBP, it is not universal. Other hypothesized mechanisms by which HBP can overcome LBBB include differential source-sink relationship during pacing compared with intrinsic conduction (due to different anisotropy ratios in the intracellular and interstitial space) and/or the virtual electrode polarization effect (in which electrical stimulus can alter refractoriness of adjacent tissue, allowing conduction in previously nonconducting tissue).[42,43]

### His Bundle Pacing after Atrioventricular Junction Ablation

The initial demonstration of permanent HBP by Deshmukh and colleagues[12] was performed in patients with refractory AF with RVR undergoing AVJ ablation. In a subsequent series of patients with AF and RVR, narrow QRS complex, and HF undergoing AVJ ablation, HBP was successful in 39 of 54 (72%) patients, resulting in an average increase in LVEF from 23% to 33% after 42 months.[44] More recent case series of HBP after AVJ ablation in patients have shown higher implant success

rate (81%–95%) and also demonstrated improvements in LVEF and LV volumes with a more significant improvement in patients with reduced LVEF before implantation.[45,46] A crossover study compared HBP with RV-only pacing in 16 patients with AF and narrow QRS after AVJ ablation and found that HBP was associated with improved interventricular electromechanical delay, NYHA score, quality-of-life scores, 6-minute walk distances, and AV valve regurgitation compared with RV-only pacing.[47] The superiority of HBP over RV-only pacing was reinforced by a recent meta-analysis that found that HBP results in higher LVEF, NYHA class improvement, less dyssynchrony, and shorter QRS duration compared with RV-only pacing as well as by a study demonstrating better clinical outcomes with HBP compared with RV-only pacing.[48,49]

### Hemodynamic Effects of His Bundle Pacing

Hemodynamic studies of HBP have shown that compared with RV-only pacing, HBP produced superior hemodynamics compared with RV-only pacing. Aortic flow and dP/dT have been shown to be higher with HBP compared with RV-only pacing and closely mirrored that seen in atrial pacing or native conduction.[50,51] In patients with a high degree of AV block and narrow QRS (<120 milliseconds), HBP resulted in higher echocardiographic acute measures of cardiac output (left ventricular outflow tract velocity time integral), and less interventricular dyssynchrony compared with RV-only pacing.[52] In addition, a study of myocardial perfusion during pacing showed that HBP results in a more physiologic blood flow compared with RV-only pacing.[53]

In pressure volume loops comparing LV hemodynamics during BiV pacing, LV-only pacing and HBP+LV pacing showed improved function compared with baseline conduction in patients with LBBB; however, BiV pacing and LV-only pacing required optimization of AV delays to achieve optimal hemodynamics, whereas HBP+LV pacing improved function at all tested AV intervals.[31] The investigators suggest that this robustness of response to AV delay is due to the ability for HBP to more effectively recruit the RV conduction system compared with BiV pacing. This effect would seemingly also favor HBP in the setting of AF given the loss of AV synchrony associated with the dysrhythmia.

### Challenges in His Bundle Pacing

Part of the explanation as to the 33-year gap between the first description of HBP and its use i a permanent pacing device in humans stems from the difficulty in securing a permanent lead that consistently allows capture of the His bundle. The development of specialized pacing leads (Select Secure 3830; Medtronic, Minneapolis, MN, USA) and delivery sheaths (C315His, C304 SelectSite; Medtronic) has been instrumental in making this technology more practically achievable in clinical practice.[54] Even with these tools,

it can be difficult to achieve selective HBP (pure His capture pacing as opposed to nonselective HBP where both the His and adjacent RV tissue is captured; **Fig. 1**); however, some studies have shown that nonselective HBP may improve ventricular dyssynchrony just as effectively as selective HBP.[55–57] HBP typically requires higher output to achieve consistent capture; however, these thresholds are typically stable during

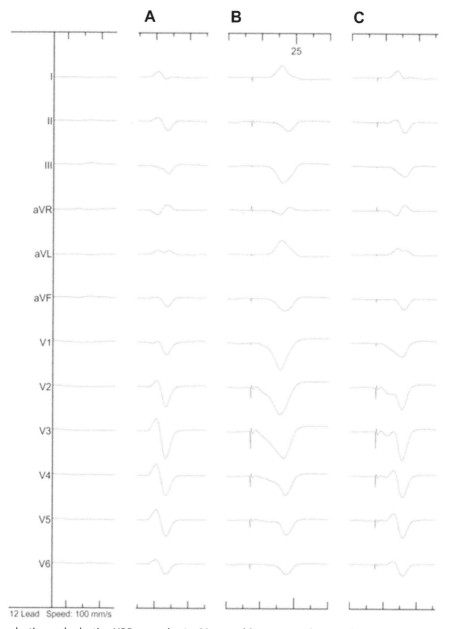

**Fig. 1.** Nonselective and selective HBP example. An 80-year-old woman with AF underwent His bundle implantation. (*A*) Native condition demonstrating a narrow QRS complex. (*B*) Pacing at high output results in nonselective His bundle capture with a widening of the QRS complex. (*C*) Selective His bundle capture with narrow QRS complex, similar to native conduction.

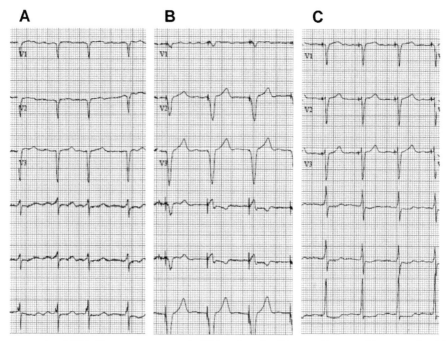

**Fig. 2.** Case example of HBP after poor response to BiV pacing. An 82-year-old man with worsening HF after BiV pacing implemented for permanent AF and heart block. (*A*) Baseline electrocardiogram demonstrated a normal QRS width of 106 milliseconds, with a nonischemic cardiomyopathy and EF of 35%. (*B*) After placement of a BiV pacemaker, the QRS width increased to 146 milliseconds with a resultant decrease in EF to 25%. (*C*) HBP pacing was implemented with selective His capture resulting in a return to a narrow QRS width of 108 milliseconds and subsequent improvement of EF to 45%.

follow-up and rarely result in premature battery depletion and early generator change.[49,58,59] Concurrent AVJ ablation presents even more challenges given the close proximity of the AVJ and optimal HBP pacing site. In fact, some operators advocate using successful HBP sites as a target to determine the optimal AVJ locations for ablation.[60] Careful monitoring of pacing threshold should be performed during ablation to avoid unwanted increases in HBP pacing thresholds during and after ablation.[46]

### Biventricular Versus His Bundle Pacing

As tempting as it may be to declare HBP the modality of choice after AVJ in patients with HF given the rather dramatic ability to preserve native physiologic conduction, the optimal pacing modality will likely be determined by many factors other than simply a desire for a narrow versus wide paced QRS morphology. Unfortunately, there are no head-to-head randomized outcomes trials comparing BiV pacemakers with HBP. The available evidence is limited with preliminary findings primarily available in the form of observational studies, and long-term efficacy and safety data are still lacking. Despite this, the preponderance of data appears to favor HBP. One such study

demonstrated that when used as an alternative CRT strategy in patients in whom BiV pacing is not feasible, HBP improved NYHA class and echocardiographic parameters.[61] A small, crossover trial (n = 12 completed crossover patients) comparing HBP with BiV pacing in a CRT-eligible population found that HBP and BiV pacing had similar effects on clinical and echocardiographic outcomes at 1 year.[62] A multicenter analysis of patients undergoing HBP after either nonresponse to BiV pacing or as a primary alternative to BiV pacing showed a high implant success rate (90%) and demonstrated significant narrowing of QRS duration, increase in LVEF, and improvement in NYHA class (example in **Fig. 2**).[63] With the improved physiologic parameters and growing body of literature, in the authors' center, HBP is often attempted first in patients with depressed EFs needing AVJ ablation. If difficulty is encountered with either lead placement or suboptimal thresholds are obtained, BiV pacing is pursued as the second option.

### SUMMARY

AF and HF are growing epidemics that share many risk factors and negatively impact one another. Although AVJ ablation with pacemaker

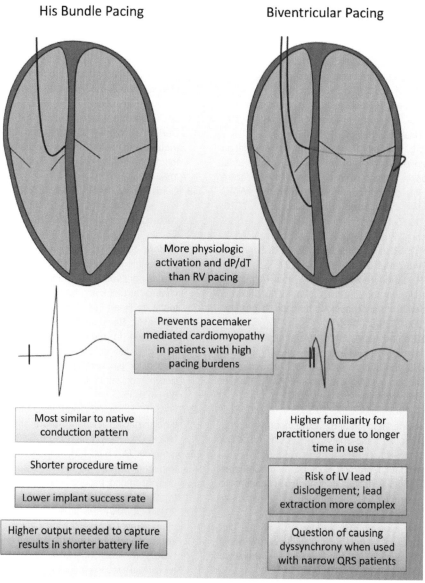

**Fig. 3.** Advantages and disadvantages of HBP and BiV pacing. Summary of the advantages and disadvantages of His bundle and BiV pacing.

implantation can be an effective strategy to achieve better rate control and improve clinical outcomes in patients with refractory AF and RVR, the choice between BiV pacing versus HBP is still not clear. HBP provides favorable physiologic electrical activation and hemodynamic profiles with shorter procedure time and no requirement for CS lead placement (**Fig. 3**). However, with His bundle lead implant failure rates still reported as high as 40%,[64] combined AVJ and HBP continues to be limited despite the positive physiologic impact of HBP. Improvements in implant technique as well as future

head-to-head clinical trials will have profound impact on management decisions in this rapidly growing population for years to come.

## ACKNOWLEDGMENTS

Dr. Loring is supported by a training grant from the National Institutes of Health T32-HL069749.

## REFERENCES

1. Patel NJ, Deshmukh A, Pant S, et al. Contemporary trends of hospitalization for atrial fibrillation in the

United States, 2000 through 2010: implications for healthcare planning. Circulation 2014;129(23): 2371–9.

2. Freeman JV, Wang Y, Akar J, et al. National trends in atrial fibrillation hospitalization, readmission, and mortality for medicare beneficiaries, 1999-2013. Circulation 2017;135(13):1227–39.

3. Tadros R, Khairy P, Rouleau JL, et al. Atrial fibrillation in heart failure: drug therapies for rate and rhythm control. Heart Fail Rev 2014;19(3):315–24.

4. Di Biase L, Mohanty P, Mohanty S, et al. Ablation versus amiodarone for treatment of persistent atrial fibrillation in patients with congestive heart failure and an implanted device: results from the AATAC multicenter randomized trial. Circulation 2016; 133(17):1637–44.

5. Marrouche NF, Brachmann J, Andresen D, et al. Catheter ablation for atrial fibrillation with heart failure. N Engl J Med 2018;378(5):417–27.

6. Chen MS, Marrouche NF, Khaykin Y, et al. Pulmonary vein isolation for the treatment of atrial fibrillation in patients with impaired systolic function. J Am Coll Cardiol 2004;43(6):1004–9.

7. Wilton SB, Fundytus A, Ghali WA, et al. Meta-analysis of the effectiveness and safety of catheter ablation of atrial fibrillation in patients with versus without left ventricular systolic dysfunction. Am J Cardiol 2010;106(9):1284–91.

8. Wood MA, Brown-Mahoney C, Kay GN, et al. Clinical outcomes after ablation and pacing therapy for atrial fibrillation : a meta-analysis. Circulation 2000; 101(10):1138–44.

9. Scheinman MM, Morady F, Hess DS, et al. Catheter-induced ablation of the atrioventricular junction to control refractory supraventricular arrhythmias. JAMA 1982;248(7):851–5.

10. Doshi RN, Daoud EG, Fellows C, et al. Left ventricular-based cardiac stimulation post AV nodal ablation evaluation (the PAVE study). J Cardiovasc Electrophysiol 2005;16(11):1160–5.

11. Merchant FM, Mittal S. Pacing-induced cardiomyopathy. Card Electrophysiol Clin 2018;10(3):437–45.

12. Deshmukh P, Casavant DA, Romanyshyn M, et al. Permanent, direct His-bundle pacing: a novel approach to cardiac pacing in patients with normal His-Purkinje activation. Circulation 2000;101(8): 869–77.

13. Moss AJ, Hall WJ, Cannom DS, et al. Cardiac-resynchronization therapy for the prevention of heart-failure events. N Engl J Med 2009;361(14): 1329–38.

14. Linde C, Abraham WT, Gold MR, et al. Randomized trial of cardiac resynchronization in mildly symptomatic heart failure patients and in asymptomatic patients with left ventricular dysfunction and previous heart failure symptoms. J Am Coll Cardiol 2008; 52(23):1834–43.

15. Moynahan M, Faris OP, Lewis BM. Cardiac resynchronization devices: the Food and Drug Administration's regulatory considerations. J Am Coll Cardiol 2005;46(12):2325–8.

16. Tanaka H, Hara H, Adelstein EC, et al. Comparative mechanical activation mapping of RV pacing to LBBB by 2D and 3D speckle tracking and association with response to resynchronization therapy. JACC Cardiovasc Imaging 2010;3(5):461–71.

17. Curtis AB, Worley SJ, Adamson PB, et al. Biventricular pacing for atrioventricular block and systolic dysfunction. N Engl J Med 2013;368(17) 1585–93.

18. Curtis AB, Worley SJ, Chung ES, et al. Improvement in clinical outcomes with biventricular versus right ventricular pacing: the BLOCK HF study. J Am Coll Cardiol 2016;67(18):2148–57.

19. St John Sutton M, Plappert T, Adamson PB, et al. Left ventricular reverse remodeling with biventricular versus right ventricular pacing in patients with atrioventricular block and heart failure in the BLOCK HF trial. Circ Heart Fail 2015;8(3):510–8.

20. Funck RC, Blanc JJ, Mueller HH, et al. Biventricular stimulation to prevent cardiac desynchronization: rationale, design, and endpoints of the 'biventricular pacing for atrioventricular block to prevent cardiac desynchronization (BioPace)' study. Europace 2006 8(8):629–35.

21. Beck H, Curtis AB. Right ventricular versus biventricular pacing for heart failure and atrioventricular block. Curr Heart Fail Rep 2016;13(5):230–6.

22. Slotwiner DJ, Raitt MH, Del-Carpio Munoz F, et al. Impact of physiologic pacing versus right ventricular pacing among patients with left ventricular ejection fraction greater than 35% A systematic review for the 2018 ACC/AHA/HRS guideline on the evaluation and management of patients with bradycardia and cardiac conduction delay: a report of the American College of Cardiology/American Heart Association Task Force on clinical practice guidelines and the Heart Rhythm Society. Heart Rhythm 2018. [Epub ahead of print].

23. Kusumoto FM, Schoenfeld MH, Barrett C, et al. 2018 ACC/AHA/HRS guideline on the evaluation and management of patients with bradycardia and cardiac conduction delay: a report of the American College of Cardiology/American Heart Association Task Force on clinical practice guidelines and the Heart Rhythm Society. J Am Coll Cardiol 2018. [Epub ahead of print].

24. Brignole M, Botto G, Mont L, et al. Cardiac resynchronization therapy in patients undergoing atrioventricular junction ablation for permanent atrial fibrillation: a randomized trial. Eur Heart J 2011 32(19):2420–9.

25. Ploux S, Eschalier R, Whinnett ZI, et al. Electrical dyssynchrony induced by biventricular pacing: implications for patient selection and therapy improvement. Heart Rhythm 2015;12(4):782–91.

26. Ruschitzka F, Abraham WT, Singh JP, et al. Cardiac-resynchronization therapy in heart failure with a narrow QRS complex. N Engl J Med 2013;369(15): 1395–405.

27. Thibault B, Harel F, Ducharme A, et al. Cardiac resynchronization therapy in patients with heart failure and a QRS complex <120 milliseconds: the Evaluation of Resynchronization Therapy for Heart Failure (LESSER-EARTH) trial. Circulation 2013;127(8):873–81.

28. Kang SH, Oh IY, Kang DY, et al. Cardiac resynchronization therapy and QRS duration: systematic review, meta-analysis, and meta-regression. J Korean Med Sci 2015;30(1):24–33.

29. Brignole M, Pokushalov E, Pentimalli F, et al. A randomized controlled trial of atrioventricular junction ablation and cardiac resynchronization therapy in patients with permanent atrial fibrillation and narrow QRS. Eur Heart J 2018;39(45): 3999–4008.

30. Strik M, van Middendorp LB, Houthuizen P, et al. Interplay of electrical wavefronts as determinant of the response to cardiac resynchronization therapy in dyssynchronous canine hearts. Circ Arrhythmia Electrophysiol 2013;6(5):924–31.

31. Padeletti L, Pieragnoli P, Ricciardi G, et al. Simultaneous his bundle and left ventricular pacing for optimal cardiac resynchronization therapy delivery: acute hemodynamic assessment by pressure-volume loops. Circ Arrhythmia Electrophysiol 2016; 9(5) [pii:e003793].

32. van Rees JB, de Bie MK, Thijssen J, et al. Implantation-related complications of implantable cardioverter-defibrillators and cardiac resynchronization therapy devices: a systematic review of randomized clinical trials. J Am Coll Cardiol 2011;58(10):995–1000.

33. Cronin EM, Wilkoff BL. Coronary sinus lead extraction. Heart Fail Clin 2017;13(1):105–15.

34. Brunner MP, Cronin EM, Duarte VE, et al. Clinical predictors of adverse patient outcomes in an experience of more than 5000 chronic endovascular pacemaker and defibrillator lead extractions. Heart Rhythm 2014;11(5):799–805.

35. Scherlag BJ, Kosowsky BD, Damato AN. A technique for ventricular pacing from the His bundle of the intact heart. J Appl Physiol 1967;22(3):584–7.

36. Scherlag BJ, Lau SH, Helfant RH, et al. Catheter technique for recording His bundle activity in man. Circulation 1969;39(1):13–8.

37. Kronborg MB, Mortensen PT, Poulsen SH, et al. His or para-His pacing preserves left ventricular function in atrioventricular block: a double-blind, randomized, crossover study. Europace 2014;16(8):1189–96.

38. James TN, Sherf L. Fine structure of the His bundle. Circulation 1971;44(1):9–28.

39. Kaufmann R, Rothberger CJ. Beiträge zur entstehungsweise extrasystolischer allorhythmien. Z Gesamte Exp Med 1919;9:104–22.

40. Narula OS. Longitudinal dissociation in the His bundle. Bundle branch block due to asynchronous conduction within the His bundle in man. Circulation 1977;56(6):996–1006.

41. Barba-Pichardo R, Morina-Vazquez P, Fernandez-Gomez JM, et al. Permanent His-bundle pacing: seeking physiological ventricular pacing. Europace 2010;12(4):527–33.

42. Vijayaraman P, Naperkowski A, Ellenbogen KA, et al. Electrophysiologic insights into site of atrioventricular block: lessons from permanent his bundle pacing. JACC Clin Electrophysiol 2015;1(6):571–81.

43. Sepulveda NG, Roth BJ, Wikswo JP Jr. Current injection into a two-dimensional anisotropic bidomain. Biophys J 1989;55(5):987–99.

44. Deshmukh PM, Romanyshyn M. Direct His-bundle pacing: present and future. Pacing Clin Electrophysiol 2004;27(6 Pt 2):862–70.

45. Huang W, Su L, Wu S, et al. Benefits of permanent his bundle pacing combined with atrioventricular node ablation in atrial fibrillation patients with heart failure with both preserved and reduced left ventricular ejection fraction. J Am Heart Assoc 2017;6(4) [pii:e005309].

46. Vijayaraman P, Subzposh FA, Naperkowski A. Atrioventricular node ablation and His bundle pacing. Europace 2017;19(suppl_4):iv10–6.

47. Occhetta E, Bortnik M, Magnani A, et al. Prevention of ventricular desynchronization by permanent para-Hisian pacing after atrioventricular node ablation in chronic atrial fibrillation: a crossover, blinded, randomized study versus apical right ventricular pacing. J Am Coll Cardiol 2006;47(10): 1938–45.

48. Yu Z, Chen R, Su Y, et al. Integrative and quantitive evaluation of the efficacy of his bundle related pacing in comparison with conventional right ventricular pacing: a meta-analysis. BMC Cardiovasc Disord 2017;17(1):221.

49. Abdelrahman M, Subzposh FA, Beer D, et al. Clinical outcomes of his bundle pacing compared to right ventricular pacing. J Am Coll Cardiol 2018; 71(20):2319–30.

50. Kosowsky BD, Scherlag BJ, Damato AN. Re-evaluation of the atrial contribution to ventricular function: study using His bundle pacing. Am J Cardiol 1968; 21(4):518–24.

51. Mabo P, Scherlag BJ, Munsif A, et al. A technique for stable His-bundle recording and pacing: electrophysiological and hemodynamic correlates. Pacing Clin Electrophysiol 1995;18(10):1894–901.

52. Kronborg MB, Poulsen SH, Mortensen PT, et al. Left ventricular performance during para-His pacing in patients with high-grade atrioventricular block: an acute study. Europace 2012;14(6):841–6.

53. Zanon F, Bacchiega E, Rampin L, et al. Direct His bundle pacing preserves coronary perfusion compared with right ventricular apical pacing: a

prospective, cross-over mid-term study. Europace 2008;10(5):580–7.

54. Gammage MD, Lieberman RA, Yee R, et al. Multicenter clinical experience with a lumenless, catheter-delivered, bipolar, permanent pacemaker lead: implant safety and electrical performance. Pacing Clin Electrophysiol 2006;29(8):858–65.

55. Catanzariti D, Maines M, Cemin C, et al. Permanent direct his bundle pacing does not induce ventricular dyssynchrony unlike conventional right ventricular apical pacing. An intrapatient acute comparison study. J Interv Card Electrophysiol 2006;16(2): 81–92.

56. Upadhyay GA, Tung R. Selective versus non-selective his bundle pacing for cardiac resynchronization therapy. J Electrocardiol 2017;50(2):191–4.

57. Zhang J, Guo J, Hou X, et al. Comparison of the effects of selective and non-selective His bundle pacing on cardiac electrical and mechanical synchrony. Europace 2018;20(6):1010–7.

58. Vijayaraman P, Dandamudi G, Lustgarten D, et al. Permanent His bundle pacing: electrophysiological and echocardiographic observations from long-term follow-up. Pacing Clin Electrophysiol 2017; 40(7):883–91.

59. Vijayaraman P, Naperkowski A, Subzposh FA, et al. Permanent His-bundle pacing: long-term lead performance and clinical outcomes. Heart Rhythm 2018;15(5):696–702.

60. Kulkarni N, Moore C, Pandey A, et al. His-bundle pacing for identifying optimal ablation sites in patients undergoing atrioventricular junction ablation: teaching an old dog a new trick. Pacing Clin Electrophysiol 2017;40(3):242–6.

61. Barba-Pichardo R, Manovel Sanchez A, Fernandez-Gomez JM, et al. Ventricular resynchronization therapy by direct His-bundle pacing using an internal cardioverter defibrillator. Europace 2013;15(1): 83–8.

62. Lustgarten DL, Crespo EM, Arkhipova-Jenkins I, et al. His-bundle pacing versus biventricular pacing in cardiac resynchronization therapy patients: a crossover design comparison. Heart Rhythm 2015; 12(7):1548–57.

63. Sharma PS, Dandamudi G, Herweg B, et al. Permanent His-bundle pacing as an alternative to biventricular pacing for cardiac resynchronization therapy: a multicenter experience. Heart Rhythm 2018;15(3):413–20.

64. Bhatt AG, Musat DL, Milstein N, et al. The efficacy of His bundle pacing: lessons learned from implementation for the first time at an experienced electrophysiology center. JACC Clin Electrophysiol 2018; 4(11):1397–406.

# Atrial Fibrillation in Heart Failure
## Left Atrial Appendage Management

Christopher R. Ellis, MD, FHRS[a],*,
Arvindh N. Kanagasundram, MD, FHRS[b]

## KEYWORDS

- Atrial fibrillation • Left atrial appendage • Intracardiac thrombus • LAA

## KEY POINTS

- Left atrial appendage (LAA) ejection velocity is reduced in heart failure patients with atrial fibrillation, promoting stasis and intracardiac thrombus, which can embolize. Left ventricular (LV) thrombus can be an additional embolic source in the setting of severe LV dysfunction.
- Independent of CHA2DS2-VASc score, an elevated serum B-type natriuretic peptide level predicts an increased risk for stroke and systemic embolism in atrial fibrillation patients.
- Closure of the LAA for stroke prevention may be appropriate for many heart failure patients; however, congestive heart failure seems associated with an increased device-related thrombus risk on the Watchman device.

## BACKGROUND
### Atrial Fibrillation and Left Atrial Appendage Thrombus as Source of Stroke

Atrial fibrillation (AF) is the most commonly encountered cardiac arrhythmia. AF is associated with significant mortality and morbidity secondary to an increased risk of embolic stroke and transient ischemic attack (TIA).[1] The left atrial appendage (LAA) is a saccular, finger-like, trabeculated structure arising from the left atrium (LA) anterior to the left pulmonary veins, thought to be a nidus for thrombus formation in greater than 90% of patients with nonvalvular AF-related stroke.[2–4] The original description by Blackshear and Odell,[2] in 1996, linked clinical stroke to LAA clot in 446 rheumatic AF subjects, and 222 nonrheumatic AF subjects. Documented LAA or left atrial clot by transesophageal echocardiogram (TEE), direct operating room observation, or autopsy was seen in 254 of 446 (57%) of rheumatic AF subjects, and in 201 of 222 (91%) of nonrheumatic AF subjects. In nonrheumatic subjects (nonvalvular AF) the clot was isolated only to the LAA, whereas rheumatic subjects frequently had thrombus extending well into the main body of the LA (**Fig. 1**).

### Congestive Heart Failure and Risk of Stroke

Both AF and congestive heart failure (CHF) are found to be comorbid, with similar underlying risk factors, including hypertension, and diabetes mellitus. CHF is a common cause of ischemic stroke,[5]

Disclosure Statement: C.R Ellis – Research funding (to Vanderbilt University Medical Center) significant; Medtronic, Boston Scientific, and Boehringer-Ingelheim (Germany). He serves on the advisory board or as a consultant (<$5000/annum) for Medtronic Inc (Minneapolis, MN), Boston Scientific Inc, Atricure, Inc, and Abbott Medical Inc. A.N. Kanagasundram is a speaker at Janssen Pharmaceuticals (<$5000/annum) and is a speaker at Zoll (<$5000/annum).
<sup>a</sup> Left Atrial Appendage Program, Vanderbilt University Medical Center, 5414 Medical Center East, 1211 21st Avenue South, Nashville, TN 37232-8802, USA; <sup>b</sup> Vanderbilt University Medical Center, 1211 21st Avenue South, Nashville, TN 37232-8802, USA
* Corresponding author.
E-mail addresses: Christopher.ellis@vumc.org; cellisvandyep@gmail.com

Cardiol Clin 37 (2019) 241–249
https://doi.org/10.1016/j.ccl.2019.01.009
0733-8651/19/© 2019 Elsevier Inc. All rights reserved.

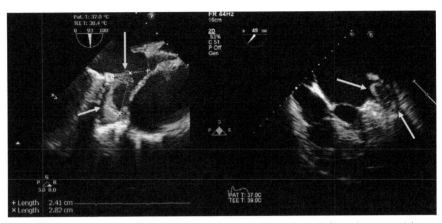

**Fig. 1.** LAA thrombus in 2 cases: left ventricular ejection fraction (LVEF) 30% (*left*) and HOCM with preserved LVEF (*right*). Yellow arrows denote LAA thrombus.

with multiple possible pathophysiologic mechanisms. AF or left ventricular (LV) hypokinesis can result in thrombus formation and a cardioembolic source[1,6] of stroke, arising from the LAA or LV cavity. A hypercoagulable state can develop due to activation of the sympathetic nervous system and renin-angiotensin-aldosterone system, leading to increased aggregation of thrombocytes and reduced fibrinolysis with increased aggregation of thrombocytes.[7] There is evidence of disordered cerebral autoregulation in patients with CHF,[8] with symptomatic carotid stenosis correlating with larger ischemic lesions in patients with reduced ejection fraction.[9] Hypotension can contribute to more extensive watershed ischemia as an additional risk factor for stroke in this population.

Data from the Framingham study indicate that the risk of ischemic stroke is 2 to 3 times higher for patients with CHF.[1] The CHADS2 score, which was validated in the National Registry of Atrial Fibrillation, revealed the contribution of a recent heart failure exacerbation toward risk for stroke. Of note, this definition of heart failure was derived from the SPAF (stroke prevention in atrial fibrillation) scheme and was a narrower definition than the currently used criteria of any heart failure. The CHA2DS2-VASc score provided a more refined estimate of stroke risk, especially in patients who had been classified as low-risk using prior schemes.[10] CHA2DS2-VASc was studied prospectively in the German AFNET registry of patients with nonvalvular AF in which one-third of the strokes or other thromboembolic events during a 5-year follow-up period occurred in patients with a CHADS2 score of less than or equal to 1. Current guidelines from ACC/AHA/ESC support the use of the CHA2DS2-VASc score. In a meta-analysis of

patients with AF and heart failure, the efficacy of novel oral anticoagulant (NOAC) regimens were shown to have significantly higher efficacy and reduced intracranial hemorrhage compared with warfarin.[11]

### Left Atrial Appendage–Emptying, Transthoracic Echocardiogram Smoke, Spontaneous Echo Contrast, Sludge, and Left Atrial Appendage Clot in Patients with Heart Failure

The development of an LAA thrombus has previously been associated with low LAA ejection velocity (LAA-EV) causing stasis of blood, with possible rouleaux formation, though a gold standard comparison to in situ thrombus or gross inspection for gelatinous clot have never been done. Computed tomography angiography and cardiac MRI are becoming frequent adjunctive imaging modalities for the LAA, which can suggest when sludge or thrombus is present in the LAA. Delayed sequence imaging (60-second delay) is essential to find late contrast filling of the LAA. The LAA may contribute to left atrial ejection of blood; however, the LAA-EV is significantly reduced in patients with systolic heart failure. Spontaneous echo contrast (SEC) and sludge seem to predict an increased risk for stroke and death on TEE imaging and are associated with both LAA-EV less than 20 cm/s and with the morphologic characteristics of the LAA. A chicken wing–shaped LAA (prominent 90-degree bend in the mid-LAA) has been associated with a lower risk of stroke in patients presenting for AF ablation and with a higher LAA-EV in TEE studies.

LAA flow pattern as maximal LAA emptying flow velocity (LAA-EV) and SEC was analyzed from 102 subjects using 2-dimensinal TEE imaging. In subjects with AF, chicken wing morphology was associated with a higher LAA emptying flow velocity (difference of means = −11.7, 95% CI 4.6–19.3, P = .003) and a reduced prevalence of SEC compared with all other LAA types (so-called non–chicken wing LAA, odds ratio [OR] 3.2, 95% CI 1.1–9.3, P = .025). This was irrespective of the phenotype of AF (paroxysmal, persistent, or permanent). Additional predictors of low LAA-EV included CHF history and an elevated B-type natriuretic peptide (BNP) level.[12] **Fig. 2** shows low-risk LAA.

The effect of elevated diastolic filling pressure on LAA-EV, formation of LAA thrombus, and SEC on TEE on 376 subjects with AF by TEE was studied by Iwakura and colleagues.[13] Diastolic filling pressure was measured as the ratio of early transmitral flow velocity (E) to mitral annular velocity (e′) on TEE. The E/e′ ratio in 28 subjects (7.4%) with LAA thrombi was higher than that in subjects without thrombus (18.3 ± 9.3 vs 11.4 ± 5.9, P <.0001). Multivariate regression analysis selected E/e′ ratio greater than or equal to 13 as an independent predictor of LAA thrombus, with an OR of 3.50 (1.22–10.61). Additional predictors of thrombus formation and SEC were LA dimension and reduced LV ejection fraction. The investigators concluded that increased diastolic filling pressure is associated with a higher rate of LAA thrombus in AF, partly through blood stasis or impaired LAA emptying function. **Fig. 3** shows high-risk LAA.

LV mass in patients with persistent AF as a marker for left ventricular hypertrophy and heart failure has also been associated with reduced LAA flow. In a case control study of 165 AF subjects, indexed LV mass and septal E′ velocity on TE, mean LAA-EV, and the presence of SEC in

the LA on TEE were predictors of thrombus. The only independent predictor of thrombus on multivariate analysis was the indexed LV mass (P<.001).[14] Atrial fibrosis has similarly been associated with lower LAA-EV and correlates with chronicity of AF and left atrial dilation, and with fibrosis associated with cardiomyopathy. Two additional TEE studies have demonstrated that TEE determination of a low LAA-EV (<20) is strongly associated with age greater than 75 years and a history of CHF (OR 2.9).[15,16] Despite a strong predisposition for LAA thrombus formation in patients with severe LV dysfunction, LV thrombus as a source of cardioembolic stroke should not be overlooked. **Fig. 4** shows LV thrombus in setting of myocarditis left ventricular ejection fraction 5% with a clear LAA.

In summary, patients with AF and heart failure are more prone to reduced LAA emptying velocity, the TEE findings of SEC, sludge, or LAA thrombus; and, through historical observational studies (CHADS and CHA2DS2-VASc score), associated increased risk of stroke and systemic embolism in AF. This is most evident in patients with persistent AF, dilated atria, increased LV mass, and increased diastolic filling pressure (**Box 1**).

## B-type Natriuretic Peptide and Atrial Fibrillation–Related Left Atrial Appendage Thrombus Risk

The definition of heart failure in the CHADS score was derived from the SPAF scheme and defined as a recent heart failure exacerbation. In contrast, the 2016 European Society of Cardiology guidelines and the definition of CHF in the CHA2DS2-VASc score attribute the added risk for CHF when "signs and symptom of heart failure objective evidence for reduced ejection fraction" are present. BNP has emerged as a powerful

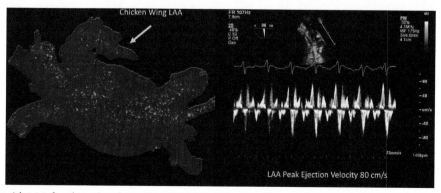

**Fig. 2.** Low-risk LAA for thrombus formation (LAA EV >80 cm/s, chicken wing morphology). Left panel CT angiogram showing LAA anatomy. Right panel TEE LAA velocity tracing (cm/s). Yellow arrow denotes chicken wing shaped LAA.

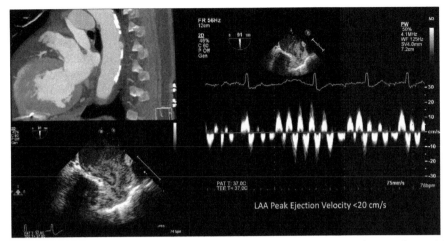

**Fig. 3.** High-risk LAA for thrombus formation (Heart failure with preserved ejection fraction [HFpEF], heavy SEC, sludge, broccoli morphology, and LAA-EV <10 cm/s). Left upper panel CT angiogram showing large windsock LAA with slow flow in distal lobes. Left lower panel TEE shows heavy 'sludge'. Right panel TEE LAA velocity tracing (cm/s).

diagnostic tool for acute heart failure exacerbation in both systolic and diastolic dysfunction. BNP is associated with LAA thrombi and the risk for systemic embolism in patients with non-valvular atrial fibrillation (NVAF).[17–19] In a prospective cohort study of subjects with NVAF,[20] high BNP was an independent predictor of thromboembolic disease and a composite of adverse cardiovascular events. BNP was shown to improve on prediction when added to the CHA2DS2-VASc score. This raises the question that BNP might be a useful biomarker, either alone or in combination with other validated scoring systems, for identifying patients at high risk for an adverse embolic event.

## Left Atrial Appendage Occlusion as an Alternative to Systemic Anticoagulation

The PINNACLE registry indicated that as many as 50% of patients with AF and a CHA2DS2-VASc score of 3 or higher were not prescribed or taking oral anticoagulation, and remained on antiplatelet agents or no therapy.[21] Five-year outcomes from the combined PROTECT-AF and PREVAIL clinical trials of the US Food and Drug Administration (FDA)-approved Watchman (Boston Scientific, Natick, MA, USA) LAA closure device support comparable stroke risk reduction to dose-adjusted warfarin (relative risk reduction ~70%) with a trend toward mortality reduction.[22] The

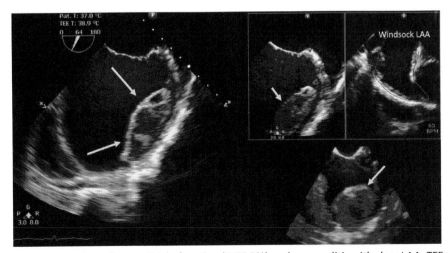

**Fig. 4.** LV thrombus in setting of severe LV dysfunction (LVEF 5%) and myocarditis with clear LAA. TEE view of LV on left panel with large LV thrombus. Right panel shows both windsock LAA and LV thrombus on TEE. Yellow arrows denotes large left ventricular thrombus.

> **Box 1**
> **Transthoracic echocardiogram findings predicting increased risk for left atrial appendage thrombus formation**
>
> - Non–chicken wing morphology
> - Reduced LAA emptying velocity less than 20 cm/s (peak)
> - Spontaneous echo contrast or sludge
> - Increased LV diastolic filling pressure (E/e' ratio >13)
> - Rheumatic mitral valve stenosis (MV area <1.5 cm$^2$)
> - Severely reduced LV ejection fraction (<30%)
> - Incomplete LAA ligation with a narrow neck
> - Increased LV mass
>
> *Abbreviation:* MV, mitral valve.

argest available data set on surgical ligation in patients undergoing open chest procedures from the Society of Thoracic Surgery database demonstrated a significant reduction in thromboembolism if the LAA was targeted for occlusion surgical LAA occlusion [S-LAAO] hazard ratio ).67; *P*<.001). Among 10,524 patients undergoing surgery (median CHA2DS2-VASc score 4), 3892 37%) underwent S-LAAO. Over a mean of 2.6 years, thromboembolism occurred in 5.4% and all-cause mortality in 21.5%. Patients undergoing S-LAAO compared with those who did not receive S-LAAO had lower rates of thromboembolism (4.2% vs 6.2%) and all-cause mortality 17.3% vs 23.9%). Patients who were discharged on anticoagulation despite S-LAAO did not obtain these benefits. However, no LAA imaging data were available postoperatively to determine if the S-LAAO was actually effective.[23]

Previous formal assessment in small randomized trials suggest as many as 30% to 40% of LAA occlusion by surgical ligation or stapled excision are incomplete. The Left Atrial Appendage Occlusion Study (LAAOS)-III clinical trial that is nearing completion will add to the data supporting LAA occlusion as a strategy to reduce stroke risk or patients with AF undergoing concomitant cardiac surgery.[24] Atriclip (Atricure Inc, West Chester, OH, USA) device placement seems associated with higher LAA closure efficacy but has not been compared with ligation in a randomized ashion.[25,26]

Patients undergoing cardiac surgery or minimally invasive valve repair who have a known history of AF and heart failure are ideally suited for considering LAA occlusion intraoperatively. The lack of a specific current procedural terminology code for surgical LAA closure and some variation in the complexity of the technique (internal vs external suture ligation, stapled excision, or placement of an Atriclip) have been barriers to adoption. Managing the LAA during cardiac surgery is particularly relevant when the patient also has a known history of LAA thrombus, intolerance to oral anticoagulation, major bleeding, or an elevated HAS-BLED score (**Table 1**).

In summary, based on observational studies of surgical LAA closure and 2 landmark randomized clinical trials with the Watchman device, LAA management (occlusion, ligation, or device closure) seems a suitable alternative to systemic anticoagulation for reduction of stroke and embolic events in patients with AF. Heart failure patients are an appealing population for consideration of LAA closure (LAAC), given reduction in LAA emptying function, and often have increased comorbidities (hypertension, end stage renal disease [ESRD], chronic kidney disease [CKD], type II diabetes mellitus, prothrombotic state, prior TIA or cerebrovascular accident [CVA]), which increase HAS-BLED scores. Alternatively, competing sources for stroke can still lead to clinical neurologic events from carotid disease, LV thrombus, and ventricular tachycardia or ventricular fibrillation arrest.

### Left Atrial Appendage Management Options for Patients at High Risk for Adverse Bleeding

Currently available surgical techniques for LAA closure include suture internal ligation, surgical excision (external ligation), GIA (Medtronic Inc, Minneapolis, MN) stapling, or clipping (Atriclip). Incomplete surgical closure from ligation or stapling seems to potentially increase the risk for thrombosis.[27,28] The Atriclip device can be placed epicardially at the base of the LAA and nonrandomized data suggest it provides highly successful occlusion (>95%)[25] with an atraumatic approach that can be achieved off-pump or via minimally invasive thoracoscopic techniques.[26] A recently published series demonstrates that salvage closure of a chronically incomplete surgical ligation can be effectively performed using the FDA-approved Watchman LAA occlusion device.[29]

Interventional percutaneous LAA closure was first reported in 2002 with the percutaneous LAA transcatheter occlusion (PLAATO) device, which was eventually withdrawn from the market in 2006. The Watchman device is the most studied LAA closure device currently in use, with 2 randomized controlled trials comparing LAA occlusion in subjects with Vitamin K antagonist (VKA)

**Table 1**
**Currently available left atrial appendage occlusion options**

| LAA Closure Approach | Composition Design | MRI Compatible | Size of LAA Approachable for Closure | Positives | Negatives |
|---|---|---|---|---|---|
| Surgical LAAO (suture ligation, stapled excision) | Typically proline for ligation GIA stapler | Yes | Any | LAA can be completely removed | LAA is often incompletely ligated, increasing stroke risk |
| Atriclip, AtriclipPRO | Titanium with woven polyester sheath, nitinol springs | Yes | Any (maximum available Atriclip 50 mm) | Excellent occlusion Electrical and mechanical isolation | May be difficult to close proximal LAA neck |
| Watchman LAAO device | Nitinol frame with polyethylene terephthalate fabric | Yes | Up to 31-mm ostium maximum | Strong clinical data High implant safety | DRT 3%–4% Frequent peridevice leak |
| Amplatzer Amulet LAA device | Distal lobe (braided nitinol mesh with 2 polyester patches) and proximal disc | Yes | 34-mm device lobe to 31-mm maximum landing zone | Can cover more complex anatomy DAPT suitable immediately | IDE clinical trial ongoing |
| LARIAT, LARIAT RS device | Ethibond (Johnson and Johnson, New Brunswick, NJ) suture on LARIAT delivery tool | Yes | Max LARIAT RS approach width 50 mm (AMAZE trial only) | No intracardiac device Electrical LAA isolation | Pericardial access a necessity Anatomic exclusions in 30%+ |

*Abbreviation:* GIA, gastrointestinal anastomosis.

therapy with subjects who have NVAF and a CHA2DS2-VASc score of greater than or equal to 1 (PROTECT-AF trial) or greater than or equal to 2 (PREVAIL trial). The combined 5-year results from these trials demonstrated a stroke prevention similar to VKA, with a reduction in major bleeding and all-cause mortality.[22] The Amplatzer Amulet LAA occluder (Abbott Medical Inc, St. Paul, MN, USA) adopts an anchor-and-seal approach with proximal device positioning allowing for placement irrespective of distal LAA anatomy. In a prospective, observational study including 1088 subjects implanted with the Amulet device, procedural success was reported in 99% with major adverse events observed in 3.2% of subjects, including major bleeding (2.4%), strokes (0.2%), and death (0.2%). The currently ongoing Amulet IDE (investigational

device exemption) trial is a worldwide prospective, randomized controlled trial designed to evaluate the safety and efficacy of this device compared with the Watchman LAA closure device.

The LARIAT RS device (SentreHEART, Redwood City, CA) is a suture delivery system that when deployed, will leave the patient with only an epicardial suture left in place, providing mechanical occlusion and electrical isolation of the LAA. A study by Lakkireddy and colleagues[3] demonstrated that the LARIAT system can lower the recurrence rate of AF in subjects undergoing AF ablation combined with LARIAT (35% vs 61%; P = .028). The prospective, multicenter US IDE AMAZE trial, which is assessing the benefit of LAA ligation in the prevention of AF in persistent AF, is ongoing (NCT02513797).

## Device-related Thrombus and Incomplete Left Atrial Appendage Closure

Device-related thrombus (DRT) can arise on the surface of any foreign body, often with the bare-metal attachment hub of the Watchman device serving as a nidus. DRT in the PROTECT-AF, PREVAIL, continued access protocol (CAP), and CAP-2 registries was reported with an incidence of 3.74%,[31] based on postimplant 45-day, 6-month, and 12-month TEE assessment (n = 65 subjects with DRT). The rate of ischemic stroke or systemic embolism in subjects with a DRT was 6.28 per 100 patient years versus 1.65 in subjects without a DRT (adjusted ratio of 3.22, P<.001). Twelve of the 19 observed embolic events occurred within 6 months of DRT detection. DRT was detected mainly at 6-month and 12-month TEE surveillance, after patients had discontinued systemic anticoagulation and were on Aspirin (ASA) 325 mg daily monotherapy. In subjects with a confirmed DRT, 16 of 65 (25%) experienced an ischemic stroke or systemic embolic event.

Individual factors associated with DRT include presence of permanent AF, increasing CHA2DS2-VASc score, larger LAA diameter, lower LAA

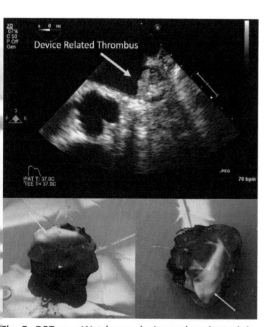

**Fig. 5.** DRT on a Watchman device and explanted device with incomplete endothelialization. Top panel TEE showing device related thrombus on Watchman device. Bottom panels show two gross anatomic views of an explanted Watchman with incomplete surface endothelialization. Yellow arrow top denotes device related thrombus on surface of a Watchman device. Yellow arrows bottom denotes small white region of complete endothelialized Watchman surface.

emptying flow velocity, and the presence of heart failure. It is probably that these are markers of a fibrotic, immobile atrium with a low-flow state and SEC in the LA. The rate of DRT was consistent with prior large European registry data, with a cumulative incidence of DRT of 2.6% at 3 months, 3.7% at 12 months, and 4.1% after 2 years.[32] Notably, patients in the EWOLUTION registry were more likely to be sent home on dual antiplatelet therapy (DAPT) only or ASA monotherapy only after implant (67%). **Fig. 5** shows DRT and an explanted Watchman device.

Several retrospective studies were published in 2017 supporting the use of NOAC or direct oral anticoagulant (DOAC) for anticoagulation post-LAA device implant to reduce DRT. The EWOLUTION registry reported a 1-year DRT rate of 3.7% with Watchman, independent of the postimplant regimen. Notably, 73% of anticoagulation-contraindicated subjects were on antiplatelet regimens alone.[33] A separate study showed a 3.2% DRT rate with the Amplatzer Cardiac Plug (previous generation of the Amulet device under IDE trial in the US).[32] When a DRT is seen, the authors' practice has been to initiate short-term oral anticoagulation and repeat the TEE in 6 weeks to ensure resolution, then return to antiplatelet therapy alone. Several trials are being designed to prospectively assess the utility of NOAC or DOAC therapy post-LAAC procedure in hopes of reducing DRT prevalence. Given the time window for when DRT was detected (most between 45 days and 6 months), perhaps oral anti-coagulation or DOAC postimplant should be continued to 90 or 180 days postimplant. Formal studies are ongoing with dabigatran as monotherapy for 90 days after LAAC (NCT03539055).

## SUMMARY

CHF contributes to an increased risk of AF-related stroke through a variety of mechanisms, both mechanical and physiologic. Anticoagulation is challenging for many patients, particularly those with higher CHA2DS2-VASc scores, and alternatives to systemic anticoagulation are needed. Clinical trials and registry data with both the Watchman LAAC device and S-LAAO support significant reduction in AF-related thromboembolic events. In addition, LAA occlusion is associated with reduced overall mortality, mainly by reducing intracranial hemorrhage or fatal bleeding. Future LAA occlusion device designs will be aimed to improve implant safety, provide a solution to challenging LAA anatomies, and reduce the incidence of DRT.

## REFERENCES

1. Wolf PA, Abbott RD, Kannel WB. Atrial fibrillation as an independent risk factor for stroke: the Framingham Study. Stroke 1991;22(8):983–8.

2. Blackshear JL, Odell JA. Appendage obliteration to reduce stroke in cardiac surgical patients with atrial fibrillation. Ann Thorac Surg 1996;61(2):755–9.

3. Leung DY, Black IW, Cranney GB, et al. Prognostic implications of left atrial spontaneous echo contrast in nonvalvular atrial fibrillation. J Am Coll Cardiol 1994;24(3):755–62.

4. Mugge A, Kuhn H, Nikutta P, et al. Assessment of left atrial appendage function by biplane transesophageal echocardiography in patients with nonrheumatic atrial fibrillation: identification of a subgroup of patients at increased embolic risk. J Am Coll Cardiol 1994;23(3):599–607.

5. Lloyd-Jones D, Adams RJ, Brown TM, et al. Executive summary: heart disease and stroke statistics–2010 update: a report from the American Heart Association. Circulation 2010;121(7):948–54.

6. Pullicino PM, Halperin JL, Thompson JL. Stroke in patients with heart failure and reduced left ventricular ejection fraction. Neurology 2000;54(2):288–94.

7. Caldwell JC, Mamas MA, Neyses L, et al. What are the thromboembolic risks of heart failure combined with chronic or paroxysmal AF? J Card Fail 2010;16(4):340–7.

8. Georgiadis D, Sievert M, Cencetti S, et al. Cerebrovascular reactivity is impaired in patients with cardiac failure. Eur Heart J 2000;21(5):407–13.

9. Pullicino P, Mifsud V, Wong E, et al. Hypoperfusion-related cerebral ischemia and cardiac left ventricular systolic dysfunction. J Stroke Cerebrovasc Dis 2001;10(4):178–82.

10. Lip GY, Nieuwlaat R, Pisters R, et al. Refining clinical risk stratification for predicting stroke and thromboembolism in atrial fibrillation using a novel risk factor-based approach: the euro heart survey on atrial fibrillation. Chest 2010;137(2):263–72.

11. Xiong Q, Lau YC, Senoo K, et al. Non-vitamin K antagonist oral anticoagulants (NOACs) in patients with concomitant atrial fibrillation and heart failure: a systemic review and meta-analysis of randomized trials. Eur J Heart Fail 2015;17(11):1192–200.

12. Kishima H, Mine T, Ashida K, et al. Does left atrial appendage morphology influence left atrial appendage flow velocity? Circ J 2015;79(8):1706–11.

13. Iwakura K, Okamura A, Koyama Y, et al. Effect of elevated left ventricular diastolic filling pressure on the frequency of left atrial appendage thrombus in patients with nonvalvular atrial fibrillation. Am J Cardiol 2011;107(3):417–22.

14. Boyd AC, McKay T, Nasibi S, et al. Left ventricular mass predicts left atrial appendage thrombus in

15. Mascioli G, Lucca E, Michelotti F, et al. Severe spontaneous echo contrast/auricolar thrombosis in "nonvalvular" AF: value of thromboembolic risk scores. Pacing Clin Electrophysiol 2017;40(1):57–62.

16. Willens HJ, Gomez-Marin O, Nelson K, et al. Correlation of CHADS2 and CHA2DS2-VASc scores with transesophageal echocardiography risk factors for thromboembolism in a multiethnic United States population with nonvalvular atrial fibrillation. J Am Soc Echocardiogr 2013;26(2):175–84.

17. Boomsma F, van den Meiracker AH. Plasma A- and B-type natriuretic peptides: physiology, methodology and clinical use. Cardiovasc Res 2001;51(3):442–9.

18. Maalouf R, Bailey S. A review on B-type natriuretic peptide monitoring: assays and biosensors. Heart Fail Rev 2016;21(5):567–78.

19. Nakamura M, Koeda Y, Tanaka F, et al. Plasma B-type natriuretic peptide as a predictor of cardiovascular events in subjects with atrial fibrillation: a community-based study. PLoS One 2013;8(12):e81243.

20. Hayashi K, Tsuda T, Nomura A, et al. Impact of B-type natriuretic peptide level on risk stratification of thromboembolism and death in patients with nonvalvular atrial fibrillation- the Hokuriku-plus AF registry. Circ J 2018;82(5):1271–8.

21. Hsu JC, Maddox TM, Kennedy K, et al. Aspirin instead of oral anticoagulant prescription in atrial fibrillation patients at risk for stroke. J Am Coll Cardiol 2016;67(25):2913–23.

22. Reddy VY, Doshi SK, Kar S, et al. 5-year outcomes after left atrial appendage closure: from the PREVAIL and PROTECT AF trials. J Am Coll Cardiol 2017;70(24):2964–75.

23. Friedman DJ, Piccini JP, Wang T, et al. Association between left atrial appendage occlusion and readmission for thromboembolism among patients with atrial fibrillation undergoing concomitant cardiac surgery. JAMA 2018;319(4):365–74.

24. Whitlock R, Healey J, Vincent J, et al. Rationale and design of the Left Atrial Appendage Occlusion Study (LAAOS) III. Ann Cardiothorac Surg 2014;3(1):45–54.

25. Ailawadi G, Gerdisch MW, Harvey RL, et al. Exclusion of the left atrial appendage with a novel device early results of a multicenter trial. J Thorac Cardiovasc Surg 2011;142(5):1002–9, 1009.e1.

26. Ellis CR, Aznaurov SG, Patel NJ, et al. Angiographic efficacy of the Atriclip left atrial appendage exclusion device placed by minimally invasive thoracoscopic approach. JACC Clin Electrophysiol 2017;3(12):1356–65.

27. Aryana A, Singh SK, Singh SM, et al. Association between incomplete surgical ligation of left atrial

appendage and stroke and systemic embolization. Heart Rhythm 2015;12(7):1431–7.

28. Katz ES, Tsiamtsiouris T, Applebaum RM, et al. Surgical left atrial appendage ligation is frequently incomplete: a transesophageal echocardiograhic study. J Am Coll Cardiol 2000;36(2):468–71.

29. Ellis CR, Metawee M, Piana RN, et al. Feasibility of left atrial appendage device closure following chronically failed surgical ligation. Heart Rhythm 2018;16(1):12–7.

30. Lakkireddy D, Sridhar Mahankali A, Kanmanthareddy A, et al. Left atrial appendage ligation and ablation for persistent atrial fibrillation: the LAALA-AF registry. JACC Clin Electrophysiol 2015;1(3):153–60.

31. Dukkipati SR, Kar S, Holmes DR Jr, et al. Device-related thrombus after left atrial appendage closure. Circulation 2018;138(9):874–85.

32. Saw J, Tzikas A, Shakir S, et al. Incidence and clinical impact of device-associated thrombus and peri-device leak following left atrial appendage closure with the amplatzer cardiac plug. JACC Cardiovasc Interv 2017;10(4):391–9.

33. Boersma LV, Schmidt B, Betts TR, et al. Implant success and safety of left atrial appendage closure with the WATCHMAN device: peri-procedural outcomes from the EWOLUTION registry. Eur Heart J 2016; 37(31):2465–74.